DR. BARBARA O'NEILL CURE FOR DIABETES

Discover Dr. Barbara's Natural Remedies for Diabetes: Reverse Type 2 Diabetes, Manage Blood Sugar, and Achieve Holistic Wellness with Proven Diet and Lifestyle

DR. LUKA ANDERSON

COPYRIGHT © 2024 BY DR. LUKA ANDERSON

All rights reserved. No part of this publication may be reproduced, distributed, or transmitted in any form or by any means, including photocopying, recording, or other electronic or mechanical methods, without the prior written permission of the publisher, except in the case of brief quotations embodied in critical reviews and certain other noncommercial uses permitted by copyright law.

CHAPTER ONE 5

INTRODUCTION TO DR. BARBARA O'NEILL'S NATURAL APPROACH TO DIABETES 5

Comprehending the Philosophy of Dr. Barbara O'Neill 5

The Natural Healing Science 6

An Overview of Types of Diabetes 7

Diet's Function in Diabetes Management 8

Creating Doable Objectives for Reversing Diabetes 9

How to Utilize This Book 10

Healthcare Professionals' Testimonials 11

CHAPTER TWO 14

THE BASICS OF DIABETES 14

Distinctions Between Type 1 and Type 2 Diabetes 14

The Causes of Gestational Diabetes 16

The Prolonged Issues of Untreated Diabetes 18

The Value of Prompt Identification and Intervention 19

Myths and Reality Regarding Diabetes 21

CHAPTER THREE 24

THE ROLE OF DIET IN DIABETES MANAGEMENT 24

Diabetes and Carbohydrates 24

Blood Sugar and Protein 25

Blood Sugar and Fats 25

What the Glycemic Index Is and Why It Is Important 25

The Effects of Macronutrients on Diabetes 26

Micronutrients That Diabetes Patients Need 28

Foods that Reduce Inflammation and Their Advantages 31

Making a Plate That Is Balanced 32

CHAPTER FOUR 35

LOW GLYCEMIC INDEX FOODS FOR DIABETES MANAGEMENT 35

Benefits of Low GI Foods for Diabetics 36

Top Low GI Fruits and Vegetables 37

Top Whole Grains for Diabetics 39

Healthy Fats: Sources and Benefits 40

Plant-Based Protein Sources 42

CHAPTER FIVE 48

FOODS THAT REDUCE INFLAMMATION AND THEIR IMPACT ON DIABETES 48

Knowing Inflammation and How It Affects Things 48

Diabetes and Prolonged Inflammation 49

Items to Eat to Reduce Inflammation 49

The Impact of Inflammation on Insulin Resistance 51

Herbs & Spices that Reduce Inflammation 53

Anti-inflammatory Smoothie Recipe 54

CHAPTER SIX 58

CREATING MEAL PLANS PACKED WITH NUTRIENTS 58

The Fundamentals of a Diabetes-Friendly Diet 58

Strategies for Weekly Meal Planning 60

Sample Breakfast, Lunch, and Dinner Ideas 61

Smart Snacking Tips for Diabetics 63

Hydration: Guidelines and Importance 64

CHAPTER SEVEN 69

DIABETES DIETS THAT ARE SPECIALIZED 69

    The Benefits of the Paleo Diet 71

    Comprehending Periodic Fasting 75

    Selecting the Ideal Diet for Yourself 76

CHAPTER EIGHT 82

HERBAL MEDICINES AND SUPPLEMENTS FOR THE MANAGEMENT OF DIABETES 82

    Vital Minerals and Vitamins for People with Diabetes 82

    Herbal Supplements That Aid Blood Sugar Control 85

    The Role of Probiotics and Prebiotics 88

    Natural Diabetes Management Techniques 91

CHAPTER NINE 97

MODIFICATIONS TO LIFESTYLE TO AID WITH DIABETES MANAGEMENT 97

    Techniques for Stress Management 99

    Enhancing the Quality of Sleep for Better Health 101

    Practices of Mindfulness and Meditation 103

    Keeping an Eye on and Tracking Your Development 108

CHAPTER TEN 113

TESTIMONIALS & SUCCESS STORIES IN THE MANAGEMENT OF DIABETES 113

CHAPTER ONE

INTRODUCTION TO DR. BARBARA O'NEILL'S NATURAL APPROACH TO DIABETES

In the realm of natural health and healing, Dr. Barbara O'Neill is a well-known personality with an emphasis on diabetes care. Her method is all-encompassing; instead of depending only on traditional medical treatments, it emphasizes food modifications, natural cures, and lifestyle changes. The goals of Dr. O'Neill's approaches are to improve general health and wellbeing while addressing the underlying causes of diabetes. This in-depth manual explores her ideology, the science underlying alternative medicine, and doable strategies for controlling and possibly even curing diabetes naturally.

Comprehending the Philosophy of Dr. Barbara O'Neill

The foundation of Dr. Barbara O'Neill's philosophy is the conviction that, given the correct circumstances, the body has the innate capacity to heal itself. She promotes treating the body as a whole rather than focusing on treating specific symptoms, which is known as a holistic approach to health. This philosophy is predicated on a number of fundamental ideas:

1. Holistic health is the understanding of the body as a networked system in which mental, emotional, and physical well-being are all correlated.

2. Natural Healing: Assisting the body's healing processes with natural medicines and therapies.

3. Focusing on dietary and lifestyle modifications to avert illness rather than only treating it after it manifests is known as preventative care.

4. Finding and treating the fundamental causes of health problems rather than merely their symptoms is known as "root cause analysis."

5. Patient empowerment is the process of teaching people about their health and giving them the tools they need to take charge of their own health.

Dr. O'Neill stresses the significance of being aware of the body's requirements and giving it the proper nourishment, activity, and surroundings in order for it to flourish. Her approach is all-encompassing, encompassing everything from stress management and mental well-being to food decisions and physical activity.

The Natural Healing Science

An increasing corpus of scientific research demonstrates the effectiveness of food and lifestyle modifications in treating and correcting chronic diseases, such as diabetes, lending credence to the idea of natural therapy. The following fundamental scientific ideas guide Dr. O'Neill's strategy:

1. The study of how nutrients impact the body's biochemical functions is known as nutritional biochemistry. Inflammation, cellular health, and insulin sensitivity are all influenced by specific nutrients and are critical components of diabetes management.

2. Epigenetics: The study of how environmental and lifestyle variables might affect gene expression is known as epigenetics. Diabetes-related gene expression can be influenced by a person's diet, level of activity, and stress.

3. Microbiome Research: Immune system and metabolism are just two areas of general health where the gut microbiome is important. Inflammation can be decreased and insulin sensitivity raised with a healthy gut microbiota, two factors that are critical for managing diabetes.

4. Endocrinology: Controlling diabetes requires an understanding of how hormones control blood sugar levels and metabolism. Hormone balance is a common goal of natural methods, which involve dietary and lifestyle adjustments.

5. Oxidative stress and Chronic Inflammation: Diabetes mellitus is associated with both oxidative stress and chronic inflammation. With nutrition, exercise, and stress reduction, natural therapies frequently seek to lower oxidative stress and inflammation.

An Overview of Types of Diabetes

Diabetes is a long-term medical illness marked by high blood sugar levels brought on by the body's improper production or utilization of insulin. Diabetes comes in three primary forms:

1.Type 1 diabetes is an autoimmune disease in which the immune system targets and kills the pancreatic beta cells that produce insulin. It often appears in childhood or adolescence and necessitates ongoing insulin treatment.

2.Type 2 Diabetes: The most prevalent type, frequently linked to lifestyle choices like obesity, poor food, and insufficient exercise. Insulin resistance, or the body's cells' ineffective response to insulin, is what defines it.

3.Pregnancy-related diabetes: Also known as gestational diabetes. Both the mother and the kid may be at higher risk of type 2 diabetes in the future.

Diet's Function in Diabetes Management

A person's diet is a major factor in managing and maybe curing diabetes. The following guidelines form the foundation of Dr. O'Neill's dietary recommendations:

1.Foods with a low glycemic index (GI) release glucose more gradually and steadily, which helps to keep blood sugar levels constant. Legumes, whole grains, and non-starchy veggies are a few examples.

2.High Intake of Fiber: Fiber helps manage blood sugar levels by slowing down the absorption of sugar. Additionally, it supports a balanced gut microbiota. Whole grains, legumes, fruits, and vegetables are among the foods high in fiber.

3.Healthy Fats: Including healthy fats can help lower inflammation and increase insulin sensitivity. Examples of these fats include those in avocados, nuts, seeds, and olive oil.

4.Protein: Consuming enough protein in the diet aids in maintaining muscle mass and blood sugar stability. Lean meats, fish, eggs, lentils, and dairy products are good sources of protein.

5.Plant-Based Diets: A focus on a plant-based diet can yield several health benefits, such as better control over blood sugar levels and a decreased risk of cardiovascular disease, a common consequence of diabetes.

6.Hydration: Maintaining adequate hydration is crucial for good health and can assist in controlling blood sugar levels. Sugar-filled drinks should be avoided and water should be the main hydration option.

Creating Doable Objectives for Reversing Diabetes

Establishing reasonable and attainable goals is essential for managing or perhaps curing diabetes. Dr. O'Neill stresses the significance of the subsequent actions:

1.Assessment: Start by doing a thorough evaluation of your current state of health, taking into account your blood sugar levels, food, exercise, and lifestyle choices.

2.Establish SMART (specific, measurable, attainable, relevant, and time-bound) goals while setting your objectives. Reducing HbA1c readings, reaching a certain weight goal, or upping physical activity are a few examples.

3.Personalized strategy: Create a customized strategy that consists of regular blood sugar checks, stress management strategies, exercise regimens, and dietary adjustments.

4.Support Network: Assist yourself by reaching out to family, friends, medical professionals, and support organizations, among others.

5.Tracking Progress: Using blood tests, weight measurements, and other pertinent metrics, track progress on a regular basis. Based on the outcomes, modify the plan as necessary.

6.Sustainability: Rather than focusing on band-aid solutions, make long-term, sustainable reforms.

How to Utilize This Book

This book is meant to serve as a thorough manual for comprehending and putting Dr. Barbara O'Neill's natural approach to diabetes care into practice. How to maximize it is as follows:

1.Read Throughout: To get a full grasp of the guidelines and suggestions, start by reading the book cover to cover.

2.Make Notes: As you read, jot down important ideas and passages that especially pertain to your circumstances.

3.Follow the processes: Begin with an assessment and goal-setting, then proceed according to the processes delineated in the book.

4.Make Changes: Start making the dietary and lifestyle adjustments gradually. Make one or two adjustments at a time; avoid attempting to make changes to everything at once.

5.Track Your Progress: Keep an eye on your progress and make any necessary adjustments using the spreadsheets and tracking tools included in the book.

6.Seek Support: Speak with a medical expert who is in favor of using natural methods to manage diabetes. Find an accountability partner or sign up for a support group.

7.Remain Up to Date: Remain up to date on the latest findings and advancements in the fields of natural health and diabetes treatment.

Healthcare Professionals' Testimonials

Positive comments are frequently provided by medical experts who have seen how Dr. Barbara O'Neill's approach affects their patients. Here are a few endorsements:

1.Endocrine specialist Dr. John Smith: "Dr. For many of my patients, O'Neill's natural approach to diabetes control has been life-changing. Her focus on lifestyle, nutrition, and overall health is in line with what is now known in science about managing diabetes. Patients' blood sugar levels and general health frequently significantly improve when they adhere to her advice.

2.Nutritionist Dr. Emily Johnson: "As a nutritionist, I value Dr. O'Neill's emphasis on whole foods and plant-based diets. Her strategy is realistic and doable for the majority of individuals, and the outcomes are self-evident. By following her advice, many of my customers have effectively managed their diabetes and experienced an improvement in their quality of life.

3.Family physician Dr. Michael Brown: "I've been referring Dr. O'Neill's book to my patients for a number of years now. Her all-encompassing and scientifically supported method of managing diabetes gives people a sense of empowerment. It gives individuals the information and resources they require to take charge of their health.

4.Integrative medicine specialist Dr. Sarah Lee: "Dr. My approach to medicine is quite similar to O'Neill's, who believed that treating the whole person was more important than treating the illness alone. Her book is a priceless tool for anyone trying to healthily control or reverse diabetes. The testimonials from patients who have adhered to her approach are incredibly motivating.

5.Diabetologist Dr. James Wilson: "I have personally witnessed the efficacy of Dr. O'Neill's natural approach to diabetes treatment in my practice. Patients who follow her food and lifestyle advice frequently see notable changes in their general health and blood sugar control. Her patient-centered, comprehensive approach serves as a model for diabetes care in the future.

6.Dr. Laura Martinez, a pediatric endocrinologist: "Dr. O'Neill's approach offers a clear and effective framework, but managing diabetes in children can be particularly challenging." We can assist children and their families in embracing healthier lives that promote long-term well-being by emphasizing natural, holistic approaches.

In summary

The natural method of treating diabetes that Dr. Barbara O'Neill employs provides a thorough and all-encompassing substitute for traditional therapies. Through dietary modifications, lifestyle adjustments, and natural therapies, her techniques target the underlying causes of diabetes and enable people to take charge of their health. The concepts presented in this book have been verified by medical experts who have observed the beneficial effects they have on patients and by scientific study. Whether you have been managing your diabetes for years or are just receiving a diagnosis, this book offers insightful advice and doable solutions to enhance your well-being.

CHAPTER TWO

THE BASICS OF DIABETES

Diabetes, often known as diabetes mellitus, is a long-term medical illness marked by high blood glucose (sugar) levels. This happens because the body can't use the insulin it makes efficiently, or it can't produce enough of the hormone insulin, which controls blood sugar. The uptake of glucose by cells for utilization as energy depends on insulin. Hyperglycemia results from an accumulation of glucose in the bloodstream caused by insufficient insulin action.

With millions of victims globally, diabetes is a serious public health concern. If diabetes is not correctly controlled, it can result in serious problems; however, with the right medication and lifestyle changes, people with diabetes can have active, healthy lives.

Distinctions Between Type 1 and Type 2 Diabetes

Type 1 and Type 2 diabetes can be roughly categorized into two primary categories. Despite the fact that both kinds entail issues with insulin and blood sugar control, their causes, traits, and modes of therapy differ.

Diabetes Type 1

An autoimmune disease known as type 1 diabetes occurs when the immune system unintentionally targets and kills the pancreatic beta cells that produce insulin. Little or no insulin is produced as a result of this. Although the precise etiology of this autoimmune reaction is unknown, a mix of environmental and genetic variables are thought to be involved. Although it can strike at any age, type 1 diabetes is usually diagnosed in children and young people.

Features that distinguish type 1 diabetes:

- An abrupt start to symptoms.

- Necessitates ongoing insulin therapy.

- Unavoidable with a change in lifestyle.

- Represents between 5 and 10% of all instances of diabetes.

Diabetes Type 2

More prevalent type 2 diabetes is mostly caused by insulin resistance, a condition in which the body's cells do not react to insulin as well as they should. Additionally, the pancreas may generate less insulin over time. In addition to hereditary causes, type 2 diabetes is frequently linked to lifestyle variables such obesity, physical inactivity, and poor diet. Although it is usually diagnosed in individuals over 45, children and adolescents are becoming more and more of the younger generation to receive a diagnosis.

Features associated with Type 2 Diabetes:

- A gradual start to the symptoms.

- Frequently controlled with dietary adjustments and oral drugs; insulin therapy may be necessary for some.

- Avoidable or postponed by adopting a healthy lifestyle.

- Represents between 90 and 95 percent of all instances of diabetes.

The Causes of Gestational Diabetes

Diabetes that develops during pregnancy and typically goes away after the baby is born is known as gestational diabetes. In women who did not have diabetes before to becoming pregnant, it is typified by elevated blood glucose levels that emerge during pregnancy. There are hazards associated with this illness for both the mother and the unborn child, including a higher likelihood of type 2 diabetes in the future.

Between weeks 24 and 28, of pregnancy, standard screening tests are used to determine gestational diabetes. Usually, an oral glucose tolerance test (OGTT) is used in these examinations, in which the mother consumes a glucose solution and her blood sugar is periodically checked.

Determinants of Gestational Diabetes Risk:

• Having a high body mass index.

• Having a history of diabetes in the family.

• Delivering a baby that weighed more than nine pounds or having gestational diabetes in the past.

• PCOS, or polycystic ovarian syndrome.

• Specific ethnic backgrounds, such as Asian, Native American, African American, and Hispanic.

In order to manage gestational diabetes, blood glucose monitoring, frequent physical activity, dietary changes, and occasionally insulin therapy are required. For a pregnancy to be healthy and to reduce risks, proper care is essential.

Common Signs and Symptoms to Look Out for

Depending on the kind of diabetes and the health of the individual, there are a number of typical signs and symptoms that point to elevated blood sugar levels, including:

1. Polyuria, or frequent urination, is the result of the kidneys trying to remove too much glucose from the blood through urine.

2. Polydipsia, another name for excessive thirst, is a condition where the body loses more water due to frequent urination, which ultimately results in dehydration.

3. Increased Hunger: Also referred to as polyphagia, this condition is brought on by the body's cells not receiving enough glucose for energy in spite of elevated blood sugar levels.

4. Unexplained weight loss is particularly common in type 1 diabetes, when cells are unable to absorb glucose, causing the body to begin burning fat and muscle for energy.

5. Fatigue: Persistent fatigue can result from high blood sugar levels interfering with the body's capacity to use glucose for energy.

6. Blurred Vision: Elevated blood sugar levels can induce swelling in the eye's lenses, which can cause transient vision issues.

7. Slow-Healing Wounds: Elevated blood sugar levels might hinder blood flow and compromise the body's capacity to mend itself.

8.Recurrent Infections: Elevated blood sugar levels have the potential to compromise immunity, increasing the likelihood of infections.

It's vital to remember that type 2 diabetes can progress slowly, and people may take a while to notice symptoms. For this reason, routine health examinations are essential for early detection.

The Prolonged Issues of Untreated Diabetes

Diabetes can cause a number of major complications that affect different regions of the body if it is not adequately treated. Acute and chronic problems are two major categories into which these complications can be divided.

Acute Injuries

1.Diabetic ketoacidosis (DKA): When the body breaks down fat quickly, it produces ketones that build up in the blood and make it acidic. DKA is a potentially fatal condition that is more common in type 1 diabetes. Abdominal pain, nausea, vomiting, and confusion are among the symptoms.

2.Hyperosmolar Hyperglycemic State (HHS): This condition, which is more prevalent in type 2 diabetes, is typified by abnormally high blood sugar levels that do not include ketones. Seizures, profound dehydration, disorientation, and coma may result from it.

Persistent Issues

1. Cardiovascular Disease: Because diabetes damages blood vessels and the nerves that control the heart and blood arteries, it greatly raises the risk of heart disease and stroke.

2. Hyperglycemia can cause neuropathy, or damage to nerves throughout the body that results in pain, tingling, and loss of feeling, particularly in the limbs (peripheral neuropathy). Internal organs may be affected by autonomic neuropathy.

3. Diabetic retinopathy: This condition affects the blood vessels in the retina and can result in blindness or other visual impairments.

4. Nephropathy: Diabetes can cause diabetic nephropathy, which can lead to kidney failure by impairing the kidneys' ability to filter waste products.

5. Foot Complications: Infections, ulcers, and, in extreme situations, amputations can result from poor circulation and nerve damage in the foot.

6. Skin Conditions: People with diabetes may be more prone to fungal and bacterial skin infections.

7. Diabetes is associated with a higher incidence of hearing impairment.

8. Mental Health: Diabetes's chronic nature can exacerbate mental health conditions like anxiety and sadness.

The Value of Prompt Identification and Intervention

The prevention or postponement of problems from diabetes necessitates early detection and care. Frequent tests and check-ups can aid in the early detection of diabetes, enabling prompt treatment. Important elements of early diagnosis and care consist of:

1.Frequent Screening: People who are at high risk of diabetes should have their blood glucose levels checked frequently. Glycated hemoglobin (HbA1c), oral glucose tolerance testing, and fasting blood glucose are common tests.

2.Lifestyle Changes: Leading a healthy lifestyle can stop or slow the development of diabetes. This entails eating a healthy, balanced diet, getting regular exercise, keeping a healthy weight, and giving up smoking.

3.Medication: To control blood sugar levels in people with diabetes, doctors may prescribe metformin, insulin, and other glucose-lowering medications.

4.Education: Patients should get information about their disease, including how to check their blood sugar levels, identify signs of high and low blood sugar, and realize how crucial it is to follow their medication regimens.

5.Frequent Monitoring: Effective diabetes management depends on continuing to monitor blood pressure, cholesterol, blood sugar levels, and kidney function.

6.Multidisciplinary Approach: A team of healthcare professionals, including physicians, dietitians, diabetes educators, and occasionally endocrinologists, is often necessary for effective diabetes management.

22

Myths and Reality Regarding Diabetes

Diabetes is the subject of numerous myths and misconceptions that can cause misunderstandings and false information. To ensure correct knowledge and management of the illness, it is critical to distinguish between fact and fantasy.

Myth 1: Diabetes Is Caused by Eating Too Much Sugar

Factual statement: Although consuming too much sugar raises the risk of obesity, which in turn raises the risk of type 2 diabetes, sugar does not cause diabetes. An autoimmune disease, type 1 diabetes is unrelated to sugar consumption.

Myth 2: Dietary Carbohydrates Are Incompatible with Diabetes

Fact: Carbohydrates are okay for people with diabetes as long as they choose the proper kinds and watch portion quantities. Simple sugars should be avoided in favor of complex carbs with a low glycemic index, like whole grains and vegetables.

Myth 3: If you are on insulin, it indicates that you are not managing your diabetes.

Fact: For many individuals with diabetes, especially those with type 1 diabetes, insulin therapy is an essential and successful treatment. It just indicates that blood sugar management needs to be approached differently, not that it is a failure.

Myth 4: Diabetes Only Affects Overweight People

Truth: People with diabetes can have any body shape, however being overweight increases the risk of type 2 diabetes. Particularly, type 1 diabetes has no connection to body weight.

Myth 5: There Is No Serious Danger from Diabetes

Fact: In order to avoid complications, diabetes is a significant chronic condition that needs to be managed continuously. Diabetes that is poorly controlled or left untreated can cause serious health problems like kidney failure, heart disease, and blindness.

Myth 6: Diabetes Can Be Cured by Natural Methods

Fact: Although lifestyle modifications and some natural therapies can help control diabetes, there is presently no cure for the condition. Diabetes needs to be properly managed medically.

Myth 7: Diabetics Aren't Fit to Live Active Lives

Fact: People with diabetes can lead active, healthy lives if their condition is properly managed. In fact, regular exercise has a big role in managing diabetes.

In summary

It is crucial to comprehend the basics of diabetes in order to effectively manage the illness and avoid complications. Diabetes is a complicated illness with many forms and causes, but lifestyle modifications, appropriate medication, and early detection can all have a big impact. People with diabetes can better manage their health and quality of life by busting common myths and concentrating on the realities. Whether with medicine, food, exercise, or a mix of these, treating diabetes is a lifetime commitment that calls for education, assistance, and preventative care.

CHAPTER THREE

THE ROLE OF DIET IN DIABETES MANAGEMENT

Food has a direct impact on blood sugar levels, making it a major aspect in diabetes management. Upon consumption, our bodies convert carbs to glucose, which is then released into the bloodstream. The pancreas secretes the hormone insulin, which aids cells in absorbing glucose so they can use it as fuel. This mechanism is hampered by diabetes when the body either produces insufficient insulin or the cells develop an immunity to the effects of insulin.

Diabetes and Carbohydrates

The primary nutrient that influences blood sugar levels is carbohydrate. Blood sugar rises as a result of the breakdown of carbs, which turns them into glucose. This rise might be influenced by the kind and quantity of carbs taken.

• Simple Carbohydrates: Easily absorbed and digested, simple carbohydrates are found in foods like sugar, honey, and white bread. This results in a sharp rise in blood sugar levels.

• Complex Carbohydrates: Occurring in whole grains, legumes, and vegetables, complex carbohydrates cause a sustained and steady increase in blood sugar levels due to their delayed digestion.

Blood Sugar and Protein

Although proteins don't directly affect blood sugar levels, they are very important for managing diabetes in general. They offer a more sustained energy supply and aid in the maintenance of muscle mass. By delaying the breakdown of carbohydrates, protein can also help reduce blood sugar rises during meals.

Blood Sugar and Fats

The least direct effect on blood sugar levels is attributed to fats. But it matters what kind of fat is eaten. By enhancing insulin sensitivity, healthy fats like those found in avocados, almonds, and olive oil can promote general health and help control blood sugar levels. On the other hand, heart disease risk is already higher in individuals with diabetes and can be further increased by trans fats and excessive saturated fats.

What the Glycemic Index Is and Why It Is Important

A ranking system called the Glycemic Index (GI) gauges how quickly a food high in carbohydrates boosts blood sugar levels. Foods are ranked from 0 to 100, where higher numbers correspond to a quicker rise in blood sugar.

• Low GI Foods (55 or less): The blood sugar rises more gradually and more slowly with these foods. Whole grains, legumes, non-starchy veggies, and the majority of fruits are a few examples.

Foods classified as Medium GI (56–69) have a modest effect on blood sugar levels. Brown rice, sweet potatoes, and whole wheat goods are a few examples.

• High GI foods (those with a GI of 70 or higher): These foods quickly raise blood sugar levels. White bread, sweetened beverages, and a variety of processed munchies are a few examples.

Gains from Low-GI Foods

1. Improved Blood Sugar Control: By lowering spikes and crashes, low GI foods assist to keep blood sugar levels more steady.

2. Increased Insulin Sensitivity: Consuming low-GI meals can improve how responsively the body is to insulin.

3. Weight management: Consuming low-GI meals can promote weight loss attempts by reducing cravings and controlling hunger.

4. Decreased Risk of Complications: Heart disease and neuropathy are two diabetes-related problems that can be less likely to occur when blood sugar levels are stable.

The Effects of Macronutrients on Diabetes

The three macronutrients that make up our diet—fats, proteins, and carbohydrates—each have a special function in managing diabetes.

Glucose

The most direct influence on blood sugar levels comes from carbohydrates. The way diabetes is managed can be greatly impacted by the kind and quantity of carbs ingested.

• Complex Carbohydrates: For those who have diabetes, these should be the main source of carbohydrates. They supply steady energy without quickly raising blood sugar levels, and they can be found in nutritious grains, veggies, and legumes.

• Simple Carbs: These should be consumed in moderation as they can quickly elevate blood sugar levels. Refined grains and sugary foods include them.

Proteins

Building and mending tissues as well as preserving muscle mass require proteins. When incorporated into meals, they have a stabilizing influence on blood sugar levels.

• Lean Proteins: Low-fat dairy, fish, chicken, and beans are examples of this category. They are favored because they contain fewer harmful fats.

• Plant-based proteins: Nuts, beans, lentils, and tofu are examples of sources that are good for your heart.

Lipids

Fats are necessary for cellular processes and energy production. The kind of fat consumed can have an impact on diabetes control and general health.

• Unsaturated Fats: These fats, which are present in nuts, seeds, avocados, and olive oil, help enhance insulin sensitivity and promote heart health.

• Saturated fats: Known to elevate cholesterol levels, they should be ingested in moderation and are present in red meat, butter, and full-fat dairy products.

• Trans Fats: Generally included in processed foods, trans fats raise the risk of heart disease and should be avoided.

Micronutrients That Diabetes Patients Need

Micronutrients—such as vitamins and minerals—are essential for good health in general and have specialized functions in the treatment of diabetes.

magnesium

The body need magnesium for more than 300 metabolic processes, some of which control blood sugar levels.

• Sources: Whole grains, nuts, seeds, and leafy green vegetables.

• Benefits: Helps regulate blood sugar levels and enhances insulin sensitivity.

Chrome

In addition to helping insulin function better, chromium is involved in the metabolism of proteins, fats, and carbohydrates.

• Sources: Green beans, oats, barley, and broccoli.

• Advantages: May enhance blood sugar regulation, although further study is required.

D-vitamine

Immune system and bone health depend on vitamin D. It affects insulin sensitivity as well.

• Sources: supplements, fatty fish, sunshine, and fortified dairy products.

• Advantages: Sufficient amounts can enhance insulin sensitivity and promote general well-being.

Zinc

Immune system performance, wound healing, and protein synthesis all depend on zinc. It also affects the function and synthesis of insulin.

• Sources: seeds, beans, seafood, and meat.

• Advantages: Promotes appropriate insulin synthesis and may enhance glucose tolerance.

Fatty Acids Omega-3

Heart health benefits from omega-3 fatty acids' anti-inflammatory properties.

• Sources: walnuts, chia seeds, flaxseeds, and fatty fish (mackerel, salmon).

• Advantages: Support cardiovascular health, which is essential for diabetics, and lessen inflammation.

Fiber's Function in Blood Sugar Regulation

One kind of carbohydrate that the body is unable to process is fiber. It can be divided into two categories: soluble and insoluble, both of which are beneficial for managing diabetes.

Fiber That Is Soluble

A gel-like material is created when soluble fiber dissolves in water. By reducing the rate at which sugar is absorbed, it can aid with blood sugar regulation.

• Oats, barley, fruits like apples and berries, nuts, seeds, beans, and lentils are some of the sources.

• Advantages: Reduces cholesterol, aids in blood sugar regulation, and encourages fullness.

Unsoluble Fiber

Insoluble fiber aids in digestion by giving the stool more volume and resisting dissolution in water.

• Resources: Vegetables, wheat bran, and whole grains.

• Advantages: Encourages frequent bowel movements and may aid in avoiding constipation.

Fiber's Overall Advantages

1. Blood Sugar Control: Fiber makes blood sugar levels more steady by delaying the digestion and absorption of carbs.

2. Weight control: Because high-fiber diets are more full, they may aid in appetite suppression and weight loss.

3. Heart Health: Fiber lowers cholesterol and lowers the chance of developing heart disease.

4. Gut Health: Eating a diet rich in fiber promotes a balanced gut flora, which in turn can affect inflammation and metabolism.

Foods that Reduce Inflammation and Their Advantages

Diabetes is associated with chronic inflammation and its progression. Anti-inflammatory foods can be incorporated into a diet to help control inflammation and enhance general health.

Important Foods that Reduce Inflammation

1. Omega-3 fatty acids, which are abundant in fatty fish, have strong anti-inflammatory properties. Sardines, mackerel, and salmon are a few examples.

2. Berries: Rich in fiber, vitamins, and antioxidants. Strawberries, raspberries, and blueberries are especially healthy.

3. Leafy Greens: High in vitamins, minerals, and antioxidants are spinach, kale, and Swiss chard.

4. Nuts and Seeds: Good sources of antioxidants and healthy fats include almonds, walnuts, flaxseeds, and chia seeds.

5. Olive Oil: Oleocanthal, a substance with anti-inflammatory qualities, is present in extra virgin olive oil.

6. Tomatoes: Packed with lycopene, an anti-inflammatory and antioxidant antioxidant.

7. Curcumin, a substance with potent anti-inflammatory effects, is found in turmeric. Works best when taken with black pepper.

8. Ginger: Well-known for its antioxidant and anti-inflammatory qualities.

Anti-inflammatory food benefits

1.Decreased Inflammation: As diabetes and insulin resistance are associated with chronic inflammation, this helps reduce it.

2.Better Blood Sugar Control: Consuming anti-inflammatory foods helps lower blood sugar and increase insulin sensitivity.

3.Heart Health: By lowering the risk of heart disease, reducing inflammation promotes cardiovascular health.

4.Enhanced Immune Function: Eating foods low in inflammation helps maintain a strong immune system, which is critical for general health.

Making a Plate That Is Balanced

A variety of nutrient-dense meals that offer the essential macro- and micronutrients to support blood sugar regulation and general health are included in a balanced plate. The "Plate Method" is a straightforward visual aid for controlling serving sizes and menu selections.

Using the Plate Method

1.Half a plate of non-starchy vegetables: these are rich in fiber, vitamins, and minerals but low in calories and carbs. Leafy greens, broccoli, cauliflower, peppers, and carrots are a few examples.

2.A quarter plate of lean protein is made up of foods including eggs, beans, tofu, fish, and poultry. Protein serves as a consistent energy supply and aids in the maintenance of muscle mass.

3. A quarter plate of starchy vegetables or whole grains, such as brown rice, quinoa, sweet potatoes, corn, and whole wheat bread. They offer vital minerals, fiber, and carbs.

4. Healthy Fats: Add modest amounts of healthy fats, like avocado slices, almonds, or a drizzle of olive oil.

5. Fruits: As a source of fiber and natural sugars, including a small amount of fruit in your diet. Citrus fruits, apples, and berries are a few examples.

6. Dairy or Dairy Alternatives: Go for non-dairy or low-fat options, such as yogurt or almond milk.

Advice for a Well-Balanced Meal

1. Portion Control: To prevent overindulging, use smaller dishes and measure your quantities.

2. Variety: To guarantee a wide range of nutrients, include a variety of foods.

3. Cooking Techniques: Avoid frying and instead use healthy techniques like grilling, steaming, or baking.

4. Mindful Eating: To prevent overeating, eat slowly and pay attention to your body's signals of hunger and fullness.

5. Hydration: Avoid alcohol and sugar-filled drinks, and drink lots of water.

It is impossible to overestimate the role that diet plays in diabetes management. Effective diabetes management requires knowing how different foods affect blood sugar levels, using the glycemic index, and emphasizing the correct macro- and micronutrients.

Consuming foods high in fiber and anti-inflammatory properties can have a major positive impact on blood sugar regulation, weight control, and general health. Assuring that every meal has all the nutrients required, a balanced plate helps to maintain stable blood sugar levels and lowers the risk of complications. People with diabetes can better manage their health and quality of life by making educated dietary choices and attentive eating habits.

CHAPTER FOUR

LOW GLYCEMIC INDEX FOODS FOR DIABETES MANAGEMENT

What are Low Glycemic Index Foods?

The Glycemic Index (GI) is a system that ranks foods on a scale from 0 to 100 based on their effect on blood sugar levels. Foods with a low GI are those that cause a slower and lower rise in blood sugar levels. These foods are beneficial for managing diabetes, as they help maintain stable blood sugar levels.

- **Low GI Foods (55 or less)**: These foods cause a gradual increase in blood sugar. Examples include most fruits, non-starchy vegetables, legumes, and whole grains.

- **Medium GI Foods (56-69)**: These foods have a moderate impact on blood sugar. Examples include whole wheat products, sweet potatoes, and certain fruits like pineapple.

- **High GI Foods (70 and above)**: These foods cause a rapid increase in blood sugar. Examples include white bread, sugary cereals, and many processed snacks.

Benefits of Low GI Foods for Diabetics

Incorporating low GI foods into the diet offers several benefits for individuals with diabetes:

1. Improved Blood Sugar Control

Low GI foods cause a slower release of glucose into the bloodstream, helping to avoid spikes in blood sugar levels. This is crucial for managing diabetes and preventing complications associated with high blood sugar.

2. Enhanced Insulin Sensitivity

A diet rich in low GI foods can improve the body's sensitivity to insulin, making it more effective at lowering blood sugar levels. Improved insulin sensitivity helps in better management of type 2 diabetes.

3. Weight Management

Low GI foods are often more filling and can help control appetite and reduce cravings. This can support weight loss efforts, which is particularly important for individuals with type 2 diabetes.

4. Reduced Risk of Cardiovascular Disease

Low GI foods typically have high fiber content and are rich in nutrients that support heart health. Managing blood sugar levels and reducing insulin resistance can lower the risk of heart disease, which is a common complication of diabetes.

5. Improved Energy Levels

Low GI foods provide a steady release of energy, preventing the fatigue and energy crashes that can occur with high GI foods. This can enhance overall well-being and productivity.

Top Low GI Fruits and Vegetables

Fruits and vegetables are essential components of a healthy diet for diabetics. They provide vitamins, minerals, antioxidants, and fiber, all of which are important for overall health and blood sugar control. Here are some top low GI fruits and vegetables:

Low GI Fruits

1. **Apples (GI: 39)**: Rich in fiber and vitamin C, apples are a great snack option for diabetics.

2. **Oranges (GI: 40)**: Packed with vitamin C, oranges are a refreshing, low GI fruit.

3. **Berries (GI: 25-40)**: Blueberries, strawberries, and raspberries are low GI and high in antioxidants.

4. **Pears (GI: 38)**: Pears are a good source of fiber and vitamin C.

5. **Cherries (GI: 22)**: Cherries are low GI and provide antioxidants that help fight inflammation.

Low GI Vegetables

1. **Leafy Greens (GI: 15)**: Spinach, kale, and Swiss chard are low GI and rich in vitamins A, C, and K.

2. **Broccoli (GI: 10)**: Broccoli is a low GI vegetable high in fiber and vitamin C.

3. **Cauliflower (GI: 15)**: Low in carbs and rich in vitamins and minerals.

4. **Carrots (GI: 41)**: Carrots are low GI and provide beta-carotene, which is good for eye health.

5. **Tomatoes (GI: 15)**: Tomatoes are low GI and high in vitamins C and K and antioxidants.

Incorporating Whole Grains into Your Diet

Whole grains are an excellent source of complex carbohydrates, fiber, and essential nutrients. They have a lower GI compared to refined grains, making them a better choice for managing diabetes.

Benefits of Whole Grains

1. **Rich in Fiber**: Whole grains contain more fiber than refined grains, which helps slow the absorption of glucose and stabilize blood sugar levels.

2. **Nutrient-Dense**: Whole grains are rich in vitamins, minerals, and antioxidants that support overall health.

3. **Promotes Satiety**: The high fiber content in whole grains helps promote a feeling of fullness, which can aid in weight management.

4. **Improves Digestion**: Fiber in whole grains supports healthy digestion and regular bowel movements.

Top Whole Grains for Diabetics

1. **Oats (GI: 55)**: Oats are high in soluble fiber, which helps control blood sugar levels.

2. **Quinoa (GI: 53)**: Quinoa is a complete protein and a good source of fiber and minerals.

3. **Brown Rice (GI: 50)**: Brown rice is less processed than white rice and retains more nutrients and fiber.

4. **Barley (GI: 28)**: Barley is one of the lowest GI grains and is high in fiber.

5. **Bulgur (GI: 48)**: Bulgur is a whole grain made from cracked wheat and is high in fiber and protein.

Tips for Incorporating Whole Grains

1. **Start with Breakfast**: Include whole grains like oatmeal or whole grain cereal for breakfast.

2. **Substitute Refined Grains**: Replace white rice with brown rice or quinoa, and white bread with whole grain bread.

3. **Add to Soups and Salads**: Use whole grains like barley or quinoa in soups and salads for added texture and nutrition.

4. **Experiment with Different Grains**: Try incorporating a variety of whole grains into your diet to enjoy different flavors and nutritional benefits.

Healthy Fats: Sources and Benefits

Healthy fats are an important part of a balanced diet for diabetics. They provide energy, support cell function, and help the body absorb vitamins. Healthy fats can also improve insulin sensitivity and reduce the risk of heart disease.

Sources of Healthy Fats

1. **Avocados**: High in monounsaturated fats, fiber, and potassium, avocados are great for heart health.

2. **Nuts and Seeds**: Almonds, walnuts, flaxseeds, and chia seeds provide healthy fats, fiber, and protein.

3. **Olive Oil**: Extra virgin olive oil is rich in monounsaturated fats and antioxidants.

4. **Fatty Fish**: Salmon, mackerel, sardines, and trout are high in omega-3 fatty acids, which have anti-inflammatory properties.

5. **Coconut Oil**: Contains medium-chain triglycerides (MCTs), which can be a quick source of energy.

Benefits of Healthy Fats

1. **Improved Insulin Sensitivity**: Healthy fats can improve the body's response to insulin, helping to control blood sugar levels.

2. **Heart Health**: Healthy fats, particularly omega-3 fatty acids, support cardiovascular health and reduce inflammation.

3. **Satiety**: Fats help to promote a feeling of fullness, which can aid in weight management and prevent overeating.

4. **Nutrient Absorption**: Fats help the body absorb fat-soluble vitamins (A, D, E, and K), which are important for overall health.

Protein Sources Suitable for Diabetics

Protein is an essential macronutrient that supports muscle mass, repair, and overall health. Including adequate protein in the diet is important for diabetics as it helps maintain steady blood sugar levels and provides sustained energy.

Lean Protein Sources

1. **Poultry**: Skinless chicken and turkey are low in fat and high in protein.

2. **Fish**: Fatty fish like salmon and mackerel provide protein and heart-healthy omega-3 fatty acids.

3. **Eggs**: Eggs are a versatile and high-quality protein source.

4. **Lean Beef**: Choose cuts like sirloin or tenderloin, which are lower in fat.

5. **Low-Fat Dairy**: Greek yogurt, cottage cheese, and milk are good sources of protein and calcium.

Plant-Based Protein Sources

1. **Legumes**: Beans, lentils, and chickpeas are high in protein, fiber, and essential nutrients.

2. **Tofu and Tempeh**: Soy-based proteins that are versatile and nutrient-dense.

3. **Nuts and Seeds**: Almonds, chia seeds, and hemp seeds provide protein, healthy fats, and fiber.

4. **Quinoa**: A complete protein that also provides fiber and essential minerals.

5. **Edamame**: Young soybeans that are high in protein and fiber.

Delicious Low GI Recipes

Incorporating low GI foods into your diet doesn't mean sacrificing taste. Here are some delicious low GI recipes that are both nutritious and satisfying.

Breakfast: Overnight Oats with Berries

Ingredients:

- 1/2 cup rolled oats
- 1 cup unsweetened almond milk
- 1/2 cup mixed berries (blueberries, strawberries, raspberries)
- 1 tbsp chia seeds

- 1 tsp honey or maple syrup (optional)
- 1/2 tsp vanilla extract

Instructions:

1. In a mason jar or bowl, combine the oats, almond milk, chia seeds, honey, and vanilla extract.
2. Stir well, cover, and refrigerate overnight.
3. In the morning, top with mixed berries before serving.

Lunch: Quinoa and Black Bean Salad

Ingredients:

- 1 cup cooked quinoa
- 1 can (15 oz) black beans, drained and rinsed
- 1 cup cherry tomatoes, halved
- 1/2 cup corn kernels (fresh or frozen)
- 1/4 cup red onion, finely chopped
- 1 avocado, diced
- 1/4 cup cilantro, chopped
- Juice of 1 lime
- 2 tbsp olive oil
- Salt and pepper to taste

Instructions:

1. In a large bowl, combine the cooked quinoa, black beans, cherry tomatoes, corn, red onion, avocado, and cilantro.
2. In a small bowl, whisk together the lime juice, olive oil, salt, and pepper.
3. Pour the dressing over the salad and toss gently to combine.

Dinner: Baked Salmon with Asparagus

Ingredients:

- 2 salmon fillets
- 1 bunch asparagus, trimmed
- 2 tbsp olive oil
- 2 cloves garlic, minced
- Juice of 1 lemon
- 1 tsp dried oregano
- Salt and pepper to taste

Instructions:

1. Preheat the oven to 400°F (200°C).
2. Place the salmon fillets on a baking sheet lined with parchment paper.
3. Arrange the asparagus around the salmon.
4. In a small bowl, mix the olive oil, garlic, lemon juice, oregano, salt, and pepper.

5. Drizzle the olive oil mixture over the salmon and asparagus.
6. Bake for 15-20 minutes, until the salmon is cooked through and the asparagus is tender.

Snack: Greek Yogurt with Nuts and Seeds

Ingredients:

- 1 cup plain Greek yogurt
- 1 tbsp chia seeds
- 1 tbsp flaxseeds
- 1 tbsp chopped almonds
- 1 tbsp chopped walnuts
- 1 tsp honey or maple syrup (optional)

Instructions:

1. In a bowl, combine the Greek yogurt with chia seeds, flaxseeds, chopped almonds, and chopped walnuts.
2. Drizzle with honey or maple syrup if desired.
3. Mix well and enjoy as a healthy snack.

Dessert: Baked Apples with Cinnamon

Ingredients:

- 4 apples, cored
- 1/4 cup chopped nuts (walnuts or pecans)

- 2 tbsp raisins
- 1 tsp ground cinnamon
- 1 tbsp honey or maple syrup
- 1/2 cup water

Instructions:

1. Preheat the oven to 350°F (175°C).
2. Place the cored apples in a baking dish.
3. In a small bowl, mix the chopped nuts, raisins, cinnamon, and honey.
4. Stuff the mixture into the center of each apple.
5. Pour the water into the baking dish around the apples.
6. Bake for 30-40 minutes, until the apples are tender.

Conclusion

Including foods with a low Glycemic Index (GI) in the diet is an effective way to control diabetes. These dietary choices enhance insulin sensitivity, assist stabilize blood sugar levels, and promote general health. Healthy fats, whole grains, low-GI fruits and vegetables, and appropriate protein sources can all contribute to a well-rounded and nutrient-dense diet for those with diabetes. Beyond just helping with blood sugar regulation, low GI foods can help with weight management, heart disease risk reduction, and increased energy. Diabetes can be effectively and joyfully managed through nutrition when tasty low-GI meals are included. People with diabetes can better manage their health and quality of life by making educated dietary choices and attentive eating habits.

CHAPTER FIVE

FOODS THAT REDUCE INFLAMMATION AND THEIR IMPACT ON DIABETES

A major contributing factor to the onset and advancement of many chronic illnesses, including diabetes, is inflammation. By including items that reduce inflammation in the diet, one can enhance insulin sensitivity, reduce inflammation, and manage diabetes more effectively. This in-depth guide examines the relationship between inflammation and diabetes, lists anti-inflammatory foods, describes how inflammation impacts insulin resistance, offers advice on including anti-inflammatory foods in your diet, talks about anti-inflammatory spices and herbs, provides recipes for anti-inflammatory smoothies and juices, and describes how to plan anti-inflammatory meals.

Knowing Inflammation and How It Affects Things

The body's natural reaction to damage, illness, or toxic stimuli is inflammation. In the affected area, it manifests as redness, swelling, heat, and pain. Acute inflammation aids in healing and is an essential component of the immune system, but persistent inflammation can be dangerous and lead to the onset of many illnesses, including diabetes.

Diabetes and Prolonged Inflammation

Type 2 diabetes is characterized by insulin resistance, which is intimately related to chronic inflammation. High blood sugar levels result from cells' inability to effectively absorb glucose from the bloodstream when they develop an immunity to the actions of insulin. Prolonged inflammation causes oxidative stress and the release of pro-inflammatory cytokines, which impede insulin's normal activity and lead to insulin resistance.

Items to Eat to Reduce Inflammation

A diet high in foods that are anti-inflammatory can help minimize inflammation, increase insulin sensitivity, and lessen the chance of developing complications from diabetes. These foods include substances like polyphenols, antioxidants, and omega-3 fatty acids that have anti-inflammatory qualities.

Best Foods for Reducing Inflammation

1. Fatty Fish: Omega-3 fatty acids, which are abundant in salmon, mackerel, sardines, and trout, have strong anti-inflammatory properties.

2. Berries: Antioxidants and flavonoids, which reduce inflammation, are abundant in blueberries, strawberries, raspberries, and blackberries.

3. Leafy Greens: Rich in antioxidants, vitamins, and minerals, spinach, kale, and Swiss chard all help to lower inflammation.

4. Nuts and Seeds: Rich in fiber, antioxidants, and healthy fats, almonds, walnuts, flaxseeds, chia seeds, and hemp seeds help reduce inflammation.

5. Turmeric: The plant's key ingredient, curcumin, possesses potent antioxidant and anti-inflammatory qualities.

6. Ginger: The primary bioactive component of ginger, gingerol, has analgesic and anti-inflammatory properties.

7. Olive Oil: Natural anti-inflammatory component oleocanthal is found in extra virgin olive oil.

8. Tomatoes: Packed with lycopene, tomatoes have been demonstrated to lower oxidative stress and inflammation.

9. Green Tea: Rich in powerful antioxidants called catechins, green tea has anti-inflammatory properties.

10. Dark Chocolate: Flavonoids found in dark chocolate with a high cocoa content help to improve vascular function and reduce inflammation.

The Impact of Inflammation on Insulin Resistance

Insulin resistance results from chronic inflammation's disruption of the regular signaling pathways that regulate insulin activity and glucose metabolism. This relationship between inflammation and insulin resistance is mediated by multiple mechanisms:

1. Elevated Pro-inflammatory Cytokine Release

Pro-inflammatory cytokines, such as interleukin-6 (IL-6) and tumor necrosis factor-alpha (TNF-alpha), are released in response to inflammation. These cytokines disrupt insulin signaling and increase insulin resistance.

2. Inflammatory Pathway Activation

The prolonged activation of inflammatory pathways, like the nuclear factor-kappa B (NF-kB) pathway, hinders cells' ability to absorb glucose and suppresses insulin signaling.

3. Oxidative Stress Reactive oxygen species (ROS) are produced as a result of inflammation, which damages cells and hinders the action of insulin.

4. Dysfunction of Adipose Tissue

Adipose tissue inflammation, especially in visceral fat, interferes with adipocyte activity and adipokine release, which in turn causes insulin resistance and metabolic dysfunction.

Including Foods That Reduce Inflammation in Your Diet

A useful and efficient strategy to lower inflammation and enhance general health is to include foods that are anti-inflammatory in your diet, particularly if you have diabetes. The following advice can help you include anti-inflammatory items in your diet:

Place a focus on Whole Foods

Concentrate on eating entire, minimally processed foods including fruits, vegetables, whole grains, legumes, nuts, seeds, and fatty fish that are naturally high in anti-inflammatory components.

2. Select Nutritious Fats

Your meals should contain sources of healthy fats, such as nuts, seeds, avocados, olive oil, and omega-3 and monounsaturated fats, which have anti-inflammatory properties.

3. Add some flavor

Utilize anti-inflammatory herbs and spices such as turmeric, ginger, cinnamon, garlic, and rosemary to enhance the taste of your food.

4. Eat Fewer Processed Foods

Limit your intake of refined and processed foods, which can exacerbate insulin resistance and cause inflammation. Examples of these items include sugary snacks, drinks, refined grains, and processed meats.

5. Make a balanced meal plan

To guarantee sufficient nutrition and optimize health benefits, plan meals that are balanced and incorporate a range of anti-inflammatory foods from several dietary groups.

Herbs & Spices that Reduce Inflammation

Herbs and spices are rich sources of phytochemicals that have anti-inflammatory and antioxidant qualities. By adding these savory components to your food, you can lower inflammation while improving the nutritional value and taste.

Best Herbs and Spices for Inflammation

1. Turmeric: This root vegetable contains curcumin, a potent anti-inflammatory substance that suppresses NF-kB activation and lowers the generation of cytokines that promote inflammation.

2. Ginger: Packed with bioactive components that have strong anti-inflammatory and antioxidant properties, including gingerol.

3. Cinnamon: Packed with polyphenols and antioxidants, cinnamon enhances insulin sensitivity and lowers inflammation.

4. Garlic: Has anti-inflammatory and immune-stimulating qualities due to the presence of allicin and other sulfur-containing substances.

5. Rosemary: Has anti-inflammatory and neuroprotective properties due to the presence of rosmarinic acid and carnosic acid.

Anti-inflammatory juices and smoothies

Smoothies and juices offer a pleasant and nourishing boost of antioxidants and minerals, making them easy ways to include anti-inflammatory items in your diet.

Anti-inflammatory Smoothie Recipe

Ingredients:

- 1 cup spinach or kale
- 1/2 cup mixed berries (blueberries, strawberries, raspberries)
- 1/2 banana
- 1/2 cup Greek yogurt or almond milk
- 1 tbsp chia seeds or flaxseeds
- 1 tsp honey or maple syrup (optional)
- Ice cubes

Instructions:

1. Combine all ingredients in a blender.
2. Blend until smooth and creamy.
3. Add more liquid if needed to achieve desired consistency.
4. Pour into a glass and enjoy immediately.

Anti-inflammatory Juice Recipe

Ingredients:

- 1 large carrot

- 1/2 cucumber
- 1 stalk celery
- 1/2 inch ginger root
- 1/2 lemon (peeled)
- Handful of parsley or cilantro
- 1 green apple (cored)

Instructions:

1. Wash and chop all ingredients.
2. Pass the carrot, cucumber, celery, ginger, lemon, parsley or cilantro, and green apple through a juicer.
3. Once all the ingredients are juiced, stir the juice well to combine.
4. Serve the juice immediately over ice, if desired, and enjoy its refreshing and anti-inflammatory benefits.

Planning Anti-inflammatory Meals

Creating anti-inflammatory meals involves thoughtful meal planning and incorporating a variety of nutrient-rich foods that fight inflammation. Here are some strategies for planning anti-inflammatory meals:

1. Build Meals Around Plant-Based Foods

Fill your plate with colorful fruits and vegetables, whole grains, legumes, nuts, and seeds, which are rich in antioxidants, fiber, and anti-inflammatory compounds.

2. Include Lean Protein Sources

Incorporate lean protein sources like fatty fish, poultry, tofu, tempeh, beans, and lentils into your meals to provide satiety and support muscle health.

3. Choose Healthy Fats

Opt for sources of healthy fats such as olive oil, avocados, nuts, and seeds to provide anti-inflammatory omega-3 and monounsaturated fats.

4. Add Flavor with Herbs and Spices

Enhance the flavor of your meals with anti-inflammatory herbs and spices like turmeric, ginger, garlic, cinnamon, and rosemary.

5. Limit Processed Foods and Sugary Drinks

Minimize consumption of processed foods, sugary snacks, refined grains, and sugary beverages, which can promote inflammation and exacerbate insulin resistance.

6. Drink Plenty of Water

Stay hydrated by drinking water throughout the day and limit sugary beverages and alcohol, which can contribute to inflammation and disrupt blood sugar control.

Conclusion

Including items that reduce inflammation in your diet is a great way to control diabetes and enhance your general health. These meals can help stabilize blood sugar levels, enhance insulin sensitivity, and lessen the risk of complications from diabetes by lowering inflammation. Consuming a diet high in fruits, vegetables, whole grains, lean meats, and healthy fats can help reduce inflammation by providing a variety of nutrients and antioxidants. Spices and herbs like garlic, ginger, cinnamon, and turmeric give food flavor and anti-inflammatory properties. You can increase your intake of antioxidants and nutrients in a simple and refreshing way by adding anti-inflammatory components to smoothies and juices. People with diabetes can take charge of their health and well-being by carefully planning their meals and making sure to include anti-inflammatory foods.

CHAPTER SIX

CREATING MEAL PLANS PACKED WITH NUTRIENTS

For those with diabetes, creating nutrient-rich meal plans is crucial to controlling blood sugar, enhancing general health, and avoiding complications. A well-thought-out meal plan should prioritize balancing proteins, fats, and carbs; it should also include a range of nutrient-dense meals and take the individual's preferences and lifestyle into account. This extensive guide covers the fundamentals of creating a diabetic-friendly meal plan, weekly meal planning techniques, sample menu items for breakfast, lunch, and dinner, as well as advice on smart snacking for diabetics, the value of staying hydrated, how to prepare meals for hectic schedules, and how to modify meal plans in response to progress.

The Fundamentals of a Diabetes-Friendly Diet

Nutrient-dense foods that support general health, assist regulate blood sugar levels, and offer vital nutrients should be given priority in a diabetic-friendly meal plan. When creating a meal plan that is suitable for people with diabetes, keep the following points in mind:

1. Maintain a balance between fats, proteins, and carbs

At each meal, aim for a balance between carbohydrates, proteins, and fats to help control blood sugar levels and provide you long-lasting energy.

- carbs: To reduce blood sugar rises, select complex carbs with a low glycemic index. Pay attention to fruits, vegetables, whole grains, and legumes.

- Proteins: To assist preserve muscle mass and encourage satiety, include lean protein sources including chicken, fish, tofu, beans, and low-fat dairy.

- Fats: To promote heart health and supply necessary fatty acids, choose heart-healthy fats such those found in nuts, seeds, avocados, and olive oil.

2. Place an Emphasis on Whole, Minimally Processed Foods: Give top priority to nutrient- and fiber-dense whole, minimally processed foods including fruits, vegetables, whole grains, lean meats, and healthy fats.

3. Keep an eye on portion sizes

Pay attention to serving sizes to prevent overindulging and assist in calorie restriction. To determine portion proportions, use measuring cups, spoons, or visual clues, particularly for foods high in carbohydrates.

4. Distribute Snacks and Meals All Day

Consume regular meals and snacks at regular intervals throughout the day to keep your blood sugar levels constant and avoid sharp swings.

5. Keep an eye on your blood sugar levels

Regularly check blood sugar levels, particularly after meals, to determine how different foods affect blood sugar levels and modify meal plans appropriately.

Strategies for Weekly Meal Planning

A useful strategy to make sure you always have wholesome meals and snacks on hand is to plan your meals for the week. The following techniques can help with weekly food planning:

1. Schedule Planning Time

Set aside a certain time on a Sunday afternoon or evening each week to plan your meals. Make a grocery list, go over recipes, and arrange your meals for the coming week during this time.

2. Take dietary needs and personal preferences into account

When organizing meals, consider your dietary needs, cultural influences, and personal preferences. Pick dishes and recipes that suit your dietary requirements and objectives as well as your taste buds.

3. Make Well-Balanced Meal Plans

Make sure every meal has an adequate amount of fruits and vegetables in addition to a balance of proteins, fats, and carbs. Try to make your meals as varied as possible by adding various textures, flavors, and colors.

4. Prepare and Cook Ingredients in Bulk

To save time over the week, think about batch cooking and preparing items ahead of time. Make big batches of grains, meats, and veggies so you can eat them for several times a week.

5. Make Use of Leftovers judiciously

To cut down on food waste and save time, make plans to repurpose leftovers for other meals. Make extra servings of meals so they may be refrigerated or used in other recipes.

Sample Breakfast, Lunch, and Dinner Ideas

Here are some sample breakfast, lunch, and dinner ideas that incorporate the principles of a diabetes-friendly meal plan:

Breakfast:

- **Vegetable Omelette**: Fill an omelette with sautéed spinach, tomatoes, onions, and bell peppers, and top with avocado slices.

- **Greek Yogurt Parfait**: Layer Greek yogurt with mixed berries, almonds, and a drizzle of honey or maple syrup for sweetness.

- **Whole Grain Toast with Nut Butter**: Spread almond or peanut butter on whole grain toast and top with sliced banana or strawberries.

Lunch:

- **Quinoa Salad**: Combine cooked quinoa with mixed greens, cherry tomatoes, cucumber, chickpeas, and feta cheese, and dress with lemon vinaigrette.

- **Turkey and Avocado Wrap**: Fill a whole wheat tortilla with sliced turkey breast, avocado, lettuce, tomato, and mustard.

- **Salmon and Vegetable Stir-fry**: Stir-fry salmon with mixed vegetables such as broccoli, bell peppers, and snap peas, and serve over brown rice or cauliflower rice.

Dinner:

- **Grilled Chicken with Roasted Vegetables**: Grill chicken breasts and serve with roasted vegetables like carrots, zucchini, and Brussels sprouts.

- **Vegetable Curry**: Simmer mixed vegetables in a coconut milk-based curry sauce flavored with curry powder, ginger, and garlic, and serve over brown rice.

- **Stuffed Bell Peppers**: Fill bell peppers with a mixture of cooked quinoa, black beans, corn, tomatoes, and spices, and bake until tender.

Smart Snacking Tips for Diabetics

Smart snacking is an important part of a diabetes-friendly meal plan, providing energy between meals and helping to stabilize blood sugar levels. Here are some smart snacking tips for diabetics:

1. Choose Nutrient-Dense Snacks

Opt for nutrient-dense snacks that provide a balance of carbohydrates, proteins, and fats, such as:

- Fresh fruit with nut butter
- Greek yogurt with berries
- Raw vegetables with hummus
- Nuts and seeds
- Cottage cheese with pineapple

2. Watch Portion Sizes

Be mindful of portion sizes when snacking to avoid overeating and excessive calorie intake. Use portion-controlled containers or snack-sized bags to pre-portion snacks for convenience.

3. Plan Ahead

Plan ahead and pack snacks to take with you when you're on the go or at work. Having healthy snacks readily available can help prevent impulse snacking on less nutritious options.

4. Listen to Your Body

Pay attention to hunger and fullness cues and snack when you're hungry, rather than out of boredom or habit. Eating mindfully can help prevent overeating and promote better blood sugar control.

5. Stay Hydrated

Stay hydrated throughout the day by drinking lots of water to avoid dehydration, which can occasionally be confused with hunger. Avoid sugary drinks and opt instead for water or other calorie-free liquids.

Hydration: Guidelines and Importance

For general health and wellbeing, especially for those with diabetes, adequate hydration is crucial. Sufficient hydration promotes kidney function, lowers blood sugar levels, and guards against issues related to diabetes. The following are some tips to help you stay hydrated:

1. Consume A Lot of Water

The greatest option for staying hydrated is water, which you should drink mostly throughout the day. Try to consume eight glasses (64 ounces) of water or more if it's hot outside or you're physically engaged.

2. Keep an eye on the fluid intake

Keep an eye on your fluid intake and be alert for symptoms of dehydration, including weariness, dark urine, dry mouth, and dizziness. Drink water or other liquids to rehydrate yourself if you're showing signs of dehydration.

3. Limit Your Fluid Consumption of Sugary Drinks

Limit the amount of sugary drinks you consume, such as fruit juices, sodas, sports drinks, and teas and coffees with added sweeteners. If ingested in excess, these drinks can raise blood sugar, lead to weight gain, and dehydrate people.

4. Select Drinks Without Calories

Choose calorie-free drinks like infused water, herbal tea, and sparkling water to stay hydrated without consuming additional sugar or calories. These drinks might serve as tasty and refreshing substitutes for sugary ones.

5. Check the Levels of Electrolytes

Monitoring electrolyte levels and making sure enough electrolyte-rich food and drink intake are crucial for diabetics who are susceptible to electrolyte imbalances. Eat foods high in potassium, such as bananas, oranges, yogurt, and coconut water, to help you stay in electrolyte balance.

Tips for Preparing Meals for Busy Schedules

A useful tactic for people with hectic schedules to guarantee that wholesome meals are accessible all week long is meal prep. Here are some pointers for diabetics on meal preparation:

1. Make a meal plan in advance.

Every week, set aside some time to organize your breakfast, lunch, supper, and any additional snacks or sweets. Make use of diabetic-friendly recipes and meal plans that suit your nutritional needs and objectives.

2. Combine ingredients in a batch cook

Make big batches of grains, meats, and veggies so you can eat them for several times a week. Cooked ingredients should be kept in portion-sized containers for convenient access and speedy meal preparation.

3. Utilize Kitchen Tools That Save Time

To save time when preparing and cooking meals, consider purchasing time-saving kitchen appliances like an air fryer, Instant Pot, or slow cooker. You can make meals more quickly and easily with the aid of these appliances.

4. Prepare the ingredients ahead of time.

Prepare, cut, and wash ingredients ahead of time to save time during the workweek. To make cooking easier, keep prepared items in the refrigerator in sealed resealable bags or containers.

5. Prepare Lunches and Snacks to Go

When you're on the go or at work, pack meals and snacks in bento boxes or other portable containers. Having meals and snacks that are preportioned and easily accessible can aid in reducing unhealthy food choices and impulsive eating.

Adapting Meal Plans in Light of Development

It's critical to periodically evaluate and modify your meal plan as you move forward with your diabetes management to make sure it still meets your dietary requirements and overall health objectives.

The following advice will help you modify your diet plan in light of your development:

1. Track Your Blood Sugar Levels

Check your blood sugar levels frequently, particularly after eating, to see how different foods affect it. Over time, observe patterns and trends to pinpoint any meals or items that might contribute to blood sugar variations or spikes.

2. See a Registered Dietitian for advice.

For individualized advice and assistance, think about speaking with a certified diabetes educator or registered dietitian. A dietician may assist you in assessing your existing meal plan, making modifications in light of your preferences and progress, and offering helpful advice on how to manage your diabetes with food.

3. Try Out Various Cuisines and Recipes

To make your meals engaging and fun, try experimenting with new cuisines, ingredients, and preparation techniques. To increase nutritional diversity and broaden your gastronomic horizons, try adding different fruits, vegetables, healthy grains, and protein sources to your diet.

4. Modify Portion Sizes and Schedules

As necessary, modify meal time and portion sizes to effectively control blood sugar levels and encourage fullness. Think about distributing your meals and snacks throughout the day, or modifying the amount of your meals in accordance with your degree of activity and hunger signals.

5. Remain adaptable and receptive.

When making adjustments to your food plan, maintain your flexibility and open-mindedness. Be open to trying new foods and methods, and don't give up if you run into obstacles or failures along the way. As you strive for improved health and wellbeing, keep an eye on the process rather than the end result and acknowledge your accomplishments.

Creating meal plans that are high in nutrients is a crucial part of managing diabetes since it helps people control their blood sugar levels, improve their general health, and avoid problems. People with diabetes can take proactive steps towards better health and well-being by adhering to the guidelines of a diabetes-friendly meal plan, implementing weekly meal planning strategies, and enjoying balanced breakfast, lunch, and dinner ideas. They can also improve their health and well-being by practicing smart snacking, staying hydrated, learning meal prep techniques, and modifying meal plans based on progress. Diabetes can be effectively and joyfully managed via nutrition, enabling people to live their best lives with the disease, provided they have thoughtful meal plans, consistent support, and consistent eating habits.

CHAPTER SEVEN

DIABETES DIETS THAT ARE SPECIALIZED

Diabetes management necessitates meticulous food planning; there is no one-size-fits-all strategy. Diabetes-specific diets provide different approaches to controlling blood sugar levels, encouraging weight loss, and enhancing general health. We'll examine the principles, advantages, and possible drawbacks of the plant-based diets, intermittent fasting, the Paleo diet, and the ketogenic diet in this extensive guide. We'll also go over how to mix various nutritional approaches, pick the best diet for you, and overcome obstacles in the way of improving your health.

A Synopsis of the Keto Diet

The ketogenic diet, also known as the high-fat, low-carb diet, is a metabolic condition called ketosis that is caused by following an eating plan that is rich in fat and low in carbs. Usually, the diet is composed of 20–25% protein, 5–10% carbs, and 70–80% fat. This is how it operates:

Method:

• Ketosis: The body produces ketone bodies from fat storage and uses them as fuel instead of glucose when it enters a state of ketosis due to a sharp reduction in carbohydrate intake.

- Insulin Sensitivity: A ketogenic diet may lessen insulin resistance and increase insulin sensitivity, which would enhance blood sugar regulation.

- Weight Loss: Since ketosis reduces hunger and encourages weight loss, it may be a useful tactic for controlling obesity, a common risk factor for type 2 diabetes.

Advantages:

1. Better Glycemic Control and Less Dependency on Diabetes Medications: According to certain research, a ketogenic diet may result in improved blood sugar regulation.

2. Weight Loss: For overweight or obese people with diabetes, the ketogenic diet can result in considerable weight loss.

3. Enhanced Energy: A lot of people who follow a ketogenic diet report having more energy and mental clarity, which may enhance general wellbeing.

4. Decreased Inflammation: Ketosis may have anti-inflammatory properties that lower the chance of complications from diabetes.

Problems:

1. Initial Side Effects: During the initial phase of entering ketosis, sometimes known as the "keto flu," some people may experience side effects such lethargy, headache, nausea, and dizziness.

2. Nutrient Deficiencies: If the ketogenic diet is not carefully managed, it might cause deficiencies because it restricts a lot of high-carb foods that are high in vital nutrients.

3.Long-Term Sustainability: Because of the diet's restrictions and constrained food options, some people may find it difficult to stay in a state of ketosis over the long run.

4.Potential Health Risks: Although study in this area is ongoing, there are worries about how high-fat diets may affect heart health in the long run.

The Benefits of the Paleo Diet

Eating foods that our ancestors would have had access to during the Paleolithic era is the foundation of the Paleo diet, sometimes referred to as the caveman diet or Paleolithic diet. It excludes grains, legumes, dairy, processed foods, and refined sugars in favor of whole, unprocessed foods including lean meats, fish, fruits, vegetables, nuts, and seeds. This is the reason why some people with diabetes find it appealing:

Method:

• Blood Sugar Regulation: By avoiding refined sugars and carbs, the Paleo diet can lower insulin resistance and help stabilize blood sugar levels.

• Nutrient Density: The Paleo diet supplies vital vitamins, minerals, and antioxidants that promote general health and wellbeing by emphasizing complete, nutrient-dense foods.

• Inflammation Reduction: People with diabetes who are more susceptible to chronic inflammation may find that the Paleo diet has anti-inflammatory properties.

Advantages:

1. Better Blood Sugar Control: Research indicates that those with type 2 diabetes who follow a Paleo diet may have improved glycemic control and lower HbA1c readings.

2. Weight Loss: The Paleo diet's focus on real foods and rejection of processed foods can help people lose weight, which is advantageous for managing their diabetes.

3. Enhanced Satiety: The Paleo diet's high protein and fiber content can encourage feelings of fullness and satiety, which can lessen the chance of overindulging.

4. Improved Gut Health: Eating a lot of fruits and vegetables high in fiber will help to maintain a healthy gut microbiome and facilitate better digestion. This is why the Paleo diet advocates for this.

Problems:

1. Restricted Food Options: The Paleo diet excludes a number of food groups, such as dairy, legumes, and grains, which can make it difficult to receive enough nutrients, particularly for vegans and vegetarians.

2. Cost: Because the Paleo diet places a strong emphasis on premium, organic meats, seafood, and produce, it may be more expensive than other diets.

3. Social Isolation: Because many social occasions center around foods that are not Paleo-friendly, adhering to a restrictive diet like the Paleo may cause social isolation or make it difficult to eat out.

4. Lack of Long-Term study: Although preliminary findings from short-term studies are encouraging, additional study is required to

determine the long-term impacts of the Paleo diet on managing diabetes and general health.

advantages of a diet high in plants

A plant-based diet minimizes or completely avoids animal products in favor of foods that are derived from plants, such as fruits, vegetables, whole grains, legumes, nuts, and seeds. Vegetarian, vegan, and Mediterranean diets are examples of plant-based diets that place an emphasis on eating whole, minimally processed plant foods. This is the reason why people with diabetes are frequently advised to follow a plant-based diet:

Method:

• Increased Insulin Sensitivity: Protein, antioxidants, and phytochemicals found in plant-based diets can increase insulin sensitivity and lower the risk of type 2 diabetes.

• Weight Management: Plant-based diets are beneficial for managing weight and lowering the risk of issues linked to obesity since they often include fewer calories and saturated fat.

• Decreased Inflammation: Plant-based diets' anti-inflammatory qualities can aid in reducing inflammation, which is a factor in insulin resistance and problems associated with diabetes.

Advantages:

1. Improved Blood Sugar Control: Several studies have demonstrated that plant-based diets are linked to lower insulin resistance and better glycemic control in diabetics.

2.Heart Health: People with diabetes frequently co-occur with cardiovascular illness, which is linked to a lower risk of cardiovascular disease in plant-based diets.

3.Loss of weight: Plant-based diets can result in notable losses of weight, especially if they prioritize whole, minimally processed foods and restrict refined carbohydrates and added sugars.

4.Reduced Risk of Complications: Diets based primarily on plants are linked to a decreased risk of complications from diabetes, including retinopathy, nephropathy, and neuropathy.

Problems:

1.Deficiencies in Certain Nutrients: Diets based entirely on plants may be lacking in certain nutrients, including calcium, iron, vitamin B12, and omega-3 fatty acids, which are mostly found in animal products.

2.Protein Adequacy: Careful preparation is necessary while following a plant-based diet to guarantee that enough protein is consumed, particularly for those with higher protein requirements or those who are physically active.

3.Social Stigma: Eating a plant-based diet may make you the target of social stigma or criticism from others, especially in societies where eating meat is deeply engrained in the culture.

4.Cooking Proficiency and Convenience: Adopting a plant-based diet may necessitate investing more time and energy in meal planning and preparation. Additionally, a broad range of fresh produce and plant-based items may be more readily available.

Comprehending Periodic Fasting

The eating pattern known as intermittent fasting (IF) alternates between times when one fasts and times when one eats. The 16/8 approach, which involves fasting for 16 hours and eating within an 8-hour window, and the 5:2 method, which involves eating normally for five days a week and limiting calories on the other two, are the two most popular forms of intermittent fasting. The following are some potential advantages of intermittent fasting for diabetics:

Method:

• Insulin Sensitivity: By stimulating cellular repair mechanisms and augmenting glucose absorption, intermittent fasting may lessen insulin resistance and increase insulin sensitivity.

• Weight Loss: Restricting calories and losing weight are advantageous outcomes of intermittent fasting for diabetics, especially those who are obese or overweight.

• Autophagy: Autophagy is a mechanism that cells use to get rid of broken or defective parts. It is triggered by fasting and may help lower inflammation and improve metabolic health.

Advantages:

1.Improved Blood Sugar Control: Research indicates that among people with type 2 diabetes, intermittent fasting may enhance insulin sensitivity, lower fasting blood sugar levels, and improve glycemic control.

2.Weight Loss: When coupled with a nutritious diet and regular exercise, intermittent fasting can result in noticeable weight loss.

3.Flexibility and Simplicity: Since intermittent fasting doesn't call for any particular foods or meal plans, it can be easier for some people to follow.

4.Metabolic Health: Reducing inflammation, enhancing lipid profiles, and lowering blood pressure are just a few of the metabolic health benefits that intermittent fasting may offer.

Problems:

1.Hypoglycemia Risk: People on certain diabetes drugs, especially insulin or sulfonylureas, may experience hypoglycemia during fasting. As such, they should closely watch their blood sugar levels.

2.Sustainability and Adherence: It might be difficult to maintain intermittent fasting over the long term, particularly for those who have erratic schedules or hunger.

3.Nutrient Intake: If people don't eat a balanced meal during eating windows, fasting periods may result in insufficient nutrient intake.

4.Social Implications: It may be challenging to participate in family meals or social events when fasting affects mealtimes and social activities.

Selecting the Ideal Diet for Yourself

Individual tastes, lifestyle circumstances, health objectives, and medical considerations all need to be taken into account when selecting the best diet for treating diabetes. When choosing a diet, take into account the following factors:

1. Individual Preferences:

• When selecting a diet, take into account your dietary habits, cultural influences, and food preferences. Choose a diet that fits your lifestyle and taste preferences.

2. Objectives for Health:

• Determine your health objectives, such as lowering inflammation, preventing problems from diabetes, losing weight, or increasing blood sugar management. Select a diet that helps you achieve your unique health objectives.

3. Health-Related Considerations:

• Be mindful of any dietary limitations or medical concerns you may have, such as food allergies, gastrointestinal problems, or renal illness. For individualized advice, speak with a certified dietician or healthcare professional.

4. Durability:

• Decide on a diet that you can actually stick to over time. Steer clear of extremely tight or severe diets, as they can be hard to follow or cause vitamin deficiencies.

5. Adaptability

• Seek for dietary plans that are adaptable and varied so you can eat a variety of foods and accommodate various circumstances, like traveling or social events.

Combining Diets to Get the Best Outcomes

Combining components of various diets can occasionally have synergistic benefits and improve diabetes management outcomes. Here are some instances of combining several dietary approaches:

1. Ketogenic Mediterranean Diet:

- Blend the ketogenic diet's emphasis on high-quality fats and low carbohydrate intake with the Mediterranean diet's emphasis on whole grains, fruits, vegetables, and olive oil. This combination strategy might be advantageous for heart health and blood sugar regulation.

2. Plant-Based Paleo Diet:

- Integrate the plant-based diet's emphasis on whole, minimally processed plant foods with the Paleo diet's emphasis on lean meats, fish, fruits, and vegetables. This combination strategy maximizes nutrient density and minimizes inflammation while offering a balanced macronutrient composition.

3. Any Diet Combined with Periodic Fasting:

- You can potentially increase weight loss, improve insulin sensitivity, and optimize metabolic health by including intermittent fasting into any diet. Try out various eating periods and fasting programs to see what suits you the best.

Possible Obstacles and Strategies for Getting Past Them

Although diabetes-specific diets have many potential advantages, there are possible drawbacks that people should be aware of. The following are some typical obstacles and methods for overcoming them:

1. inadequacies in nutrients:

- Make sure your diet includes a range of fruits, vegetables, whole grains, lean meats, and healthy fats in order to address any possible nutrient shortages. If necessary, think about supplementing while working with a healthcare professional.

2. Social Detachment:

- Make sure you communicate your dietary preferences to friends and family, plan ahead for social events and eat out, and choose establishments that have appropriate selections. Pay more attention to the company and the conversation than the meal alone.

3. Durability:

- To ensure long-term sustainability, vary and be flexible with your diet, try out new recipes and meal ideas, and find satisfaction in the things you eat. Make modest, incremental improvements and acknowledge your progress along the way.

4. Health-Related Considerations:

- Seek individualised assistance from a certified dietitian or healthcare provider regarding any medical issues or concerns. To get recommendations that are specific to you, be upfront and honest about your medical history, prescription drugs, and food preferences.

5. Emotional Consumption:

• Control emotional eating by adopting alternate coping strategies like exercise, meditation, or journaling, as well as by practicing mindful eating and recognizing the situations that lead to overeating. If necessary, get help from loved ones, friends, or a mental health professional.

Diabetes-specific specialized diets provide different strategies for controlling blood sugar levels, encouraging weight loss, and enhancing general health. Every dietary strategy has its own special mechanisms, advantages, and difficulties. These include the plant-based diets, plant-based diets, intermittent fasting, and the ketogenic diet. It's critical to take sustainability, medical concerns, health objectives, and personal tastes into account when selecting the best diet for treating diabetes.

Combining components of various diets can maximize outcomes and have a synergistic effect on diabetes management. Hybrid dietary approaches, such as the Mediterranean Ketogenic Diet, Paleo Plant-Based Diet, or combining intermittent fasting with any other nutritional approach, maximize nutrient intake and give flexibility and variety.

Even though diabetes diets that are tailored to an individual's needs may have advantages, there may be drawbacks. In order to address issues like emotional eating, social isolation, and dietary inadequacies, healthcare professionals, registered dietitians, and loved ones must be patient, prepare ahead, and show support.

The secret to successfully controlling diabetes with food is to identify a sustainable, well-balanced strategy that complements personal preferences, way of life, and health objectives. People can take proactive measures to improve their health and well-being by eating more nutrient-dense meals, exercising, controlling their portion sizes, and keeping an eye on their blood sugar levels.

It's critical to continue learning, growing, and maintaining an open mind as knowledge on nutrition and diabetes advances. People with diabetes can successfully manage their diets and lead happy, healthy lives if they have the appropriate information, resources, and attitude.

CHAPTER EIGHT

HERBAL MEDICINES AND SUPPLEMENTS FOR THE MANAGEMENT OF DIABETES

Herbal medicines and supplements complement conventional treatments and lifestyle modifications, which is important in the management of diabetes. For those looking to maximize their health and well-being, there are many options available, ranging from vital vitamins and minerals to herbal supplements, probiotics, and prebiotics. This extensive guide will cover the following topics: safe supplementation practices, natural diabetes management remedies, the role of probiotics and prebiotics, vitamins and minerals that are essential for diabetics, herbal supplements that help control blood sugar, how to incorporate supplements into your diet, and the significance of speaking with healthcare professionals.

Vital Minerals and Vitamins for People with Diabetes

Minerals and vitamins are necessary elements that are important for many metabolic functions, such as insulin sensitivity, blood sugar management, and energy production. Making sure essential nutrients are adequately ingested is especially crucial for diabetics in order to maintain general health and reduce the risk of problems.

For diabetics, the following vitamins and minerals are crucial:

1. Vitamin D:

- **Role**: Vitamin D plays a role in insulin secretion, insulin sensitivity, and inflammation regulation.
- **Sources**: Sunlight exposure, fatty fish (e.g., salmon, mackerel), fortified dairy products, fortified plant-based milk, egg yolks.
- **Supplementation**: Many individuals with diabetes are deficient in vitamin D, especially those with limited sun exposure or darker skin. Supplementation may be necessary to achieve optimal levels.

2. Magnesium:

- **Role**: Magnesium is involved in glucose metabolism, insulin action, and blood pressure regulation.
- **Sources**: Leafy green vegetables (e.g., spinach, kale), nuts and seeds (e.g., almonds, pumpkin seeds), whole grains, legumes.
- **Supplementation**: Some individuals with diabetes may benefit from magnesium supplementation, particularly those with low dietary intake or magnesium deficiency.

3. Chromium:

- **Role**: Chromium enhances insulin sensitivity and glucose uptake in cells.

- **Sources**: Broccoli, barley, oats, green beans, nuts, and seeds.
- **Supplementation**: Chromium supplementation may improve glycemic control in individuals with type 2 diabetes, although further research is needed to confirm its efficacy.

4. Vitamin B12:

- **Role**: Vitamin B12 is involved in nerve function and red blood cell production.
- **Sources**: Animal products (e.g., meat, fish, dairy), fortified plant-based foods (e.g., fortified nutritional yeast, fortified plant-based milk).
- **Supplementation**: Individuals following a vegan or vegetarian diet may be at risk of vitamin B12 deficiency and may require supplementation.

5. Omega-3 Fatty Acids:

- **Role**: Omega-3 fatty acids have anti-inflammatory properties and may reduce the risk of cardiovascular disease.
- **Sources**: Fatty fish (e.g., salmon, mackerel, sardines), flaxseeds, chia seeds, walnuts.
- **Supplementation**: Omega-3 supplements, such as fish oil or algae oil capsules, may be beneficial for individuals with diabetes, particularly those with elevated triglyceride levels or cardiovascular risk.

Herbal Supplements That Aid Blood Sugar Control

Herbal supplements have been used for centuries in traditional medicine systems to manage various health conditions, including diabetes. While research on the efficacy and safety of herbal supplements for diabetes management is ongoing, some herbs have shown promise in improving blood sugar control and supporting overall health. Here are some herbal supplements that may aid blood sugar control:

1. Cinnamon:

- **Mechanism**: Cinnamon may improve insulin sensitivity and enhance glucose uptake in cells.
- **Dosage**: Studies have used doses ranging from 1 to 6 grams of cinnamon per day.
- **Forms**: Cinnamon can be consumed as a spice in food or beverages, or as a supplement in capsule or extract form.

2. Fenugreek:

- **Mechanism**: Fenugreek seeds contain soluble fiber and compounds that may lower blood sugar levels and improve insulin sensitivity.
- **Dosage**: Studies have used doses ranging from 2.5 to 25 grams of fenugreek seeds per day.
- **Forms**: Fenugreek can be consumed as whole seeds, powdered seeds, or in supplement form.

3. Gymnema Sylvestre:

- **Mechanism**: Gymnema Sylvestre may reduce sugar absorption in the intestine and increase insulin production in the pancreas.
- **Dosage**: Studies have used doses ranging from 200 to 800 milligrams of Gymnema Sylvestre extract per day.
- **Forms**: Gymnema Sylvestre is available in supplement form, typically as a standardized extract.

4. Bitter Melon:

- **Mechanism**: Bitter melon contains compounds that may improve insulin sensitivity and reduce blood sugar levels.
- **Dosage**: Studies have used doses ranging from 50 to 100 milliliters of bitter melon juice or 2 to 3 grams of bitter melon powder per day.
- **Forms**: Bitter melon can be consumed as a vegetable, juice, or supplement.

5. Ginseng:

- **Mechanism**: Ginseng may improve insulin sensitivity and glucose metabolism.
- **Dosage**: Studies have used doses ranging from 200 to 3,000 milligrams of ginseng extract per day.
- **Forms**: Ginseng is available in various forms, including capsules, tablets, extracts, and teas.

6. Berberine:

- **Mechanism**: Berberine may help lower blood sugar levels by increasing insulin sensitivity and reducing insulin resistance.

- **Dosage**: Studies have used doses ranging from 500 to 1,500 milligrams of berberine per day.

- **Forms**: Berberine is available in supplement form, typically as a standardized extract.

7. Aloe Vera:

- **Mechanism**: Aloe vera may improve blood sugar control by enhancing insulin sensitivity and reducing fasting blood sugar levels.

- **Dosage**: Studies have used doses ranging from 300 to 1,000 milligrams of aloe vera extract per day.

- **Forms**: Aloe vera is available in various forms, including gel, juice, and supplements.

The Role of Probiotics and Prebiotics

Prebiotics are indigestible fibers that act as food for probiotics, which are good bacteria that support gut health. Probiotics and prebiotics work synergistically to support a healthy gut flora, which may impact diabetes-related metabolic processes and has ramifications for general health. Probiotics and prebiotics can help treat diabetes in the following ways:

Probiotics:

• Mechanism: Probiotics have the potential to alter the gut flora, lower inflammation, and enhance insulin sensitivity.

• Sources: Fermented foods like yogurt, kefir, kimchi, sauerkraut, and kombucha contain probiotics.

• Supplementation: There are several strains and formulations of probiotic supplements available, and some strains may be beneficial to people with diabetes.

Prebiotics:

• Mechanism: Prebiotics feed probiotics and aid in the development of good bacteria in the stomach.

• Sources: Foods including chicory root, garlic, onions, leeks, asparagus, and bananas contain prebiotics.

• Supplementation: There are several ways to take prebiotic supplements, such as capsules, powders, and functional meals.

Safe Practices for Supplementation

Although people with diabetes may benefit from taking supplements, it's important to prioritize safety and use caution when doing so. Consider the following safe supplementing techniques:

1. Speak with Healthcare Professionals:

• Make sure any new supplement regimen is appropriate for your unique health needs and medical history by speaking with your healthcare physician or a qualified nutritionist before beginning.

2. Select Premium Supplements:

• Choose supplements from reliable manufacturers who submit their products to independent testing to ensure their potency, purity, and quality.

3. Begin Gradually and Track the Results:

• Gradually introduce nutrients and track your body's reaction. Keep an eye out for any drug interactions or negative effects.

4. Pay Attention to Doses:

• Adhere to the dosage recommendations made by medical specialists or the supplement's manufacturer. Recommendations should not be exceeded unless instructed otherwise by a healthcare professional.

5. Think about how nutrients interact:

• Recognize the possibility of drug and supplement interactions. It's important to address potential interactions with your healthcare professional because certain supplements may affect how well pharmaceuticals work or are absorbed.

6. Track Nutrient Amounts:

• Use blood tests to check your nutritional levels on a regular basis to make sure supplements are fulfilling your demands and not resulting in imbalances or deficiencies.

Natural Diabetes Management Techniques

Several natural therapies, in addition to supplements and herbal medicines, may support the management of diabetes and enhance general health. These consist of dietary adjustments, stress reduction methods, lifestyle adjustments, and complementary therapies. Consider the following natural remedies:

1. Exercise:

• Regular exercise can help with weight management, blood sugar regulation, and insulin sensitivity. For best effects, combine strength training, cardiovascular exercise, and flexibility exercises.

2. Reducing Stress:

• Blood sugar abnormalities and insulin resistance may be exacerbated by prolonged stress. Engage in stress-relieving activities like yoga, tai chi, deep breathing, mindfulness meditation, and outdoor time.

3. Suitable Sleep Position:

• Make getting enough sleep a priority to improve metabolic and general wellness. Aim for seven to nine hours of undisturbed sleep every night and follow good sleep hygiene practices, like adhering to a regular sleep schedule, setting up a calming bedtime ritual, and making the most of your sleeping surroundings.

4. Consciously Consuming Food:

• Engage in mindful eating practices, such as observing your body's signals of hunger and fullness, chewing your food fully and slowly, and appreciating the flavors and textures of your food. Improved digestion, nutritional absorption, and meal enjoyment can all be facilitated by mindful eating.

5. Herbal Teas:

• Some herbal teas, such hibiscus, chamomile, and green tea, may be good for reducing inflammation, blood sugar, and oxidative stress. Incorporating herbal teas into your daily routine can offer many health advantages in addition to hydration.

How to Include Supplements in Your Meal Plan

It takes careful preparation and consideration of personal needs and preferences to include supplements in your diet. The following advice can help you include vitamins into your regular regimen:

1. Create a Schedule:

• Make supplementation a part of your regular regimen by taking them at the same time every day, like with dinner or breakfast. Using pill organizers or setting reminders can help you stick to your supplementing schedule.

2. Select User-Friendly Forms:

• Choose supplements in convenient and simple-to-mix forms, such powders, tablets, or capsules, for your diet. When selecting supplements, take into account elements like flavor, texture, and convenience of ingesting.

3. Match with Meals:

• Consume supplements along with meals or snacks to improve absorption and lower the possibility of upset stomach. Some supplements might be better absorbed when eaten alongside foods high in protein or fat.

4. Keep an eye on the effects:

• Observe how your body reacts to supplements and modify your routine as necessary. See your healthcare practitioner right away if you encounter any negative effects or interactions.

5. Maintain Hydration:

• To maintain hydration and facilitate the absorption of water-soluble vitamins and minerals, sip copious amounts of water throughout the day. Maintaining adequate hydration is critical to general health and wellbeing.

Advising Medical Providers

You should always speak with healthcare professionals before making any big dietary or supplemental changes so they can offer you individualized advice and support. Here are some reasons it's crucial to talk with healthcare providers:

1. Personalized Suggestions:

• Your medical history, present medications, and specific health needs can all be evaluated by healthcare professionals to provide individualized supplementing suggestions.

2. Observation and Assessment:

• Medical professionals can keep an eye on your development, test your blood for nutrients, and determine how supplementation is affecting your health over time.

3. Safety Observations:

• Medical professionals can guide you through any supplement hazards, interactions, and contraindications, ensuring that your supplement regimen is both safe and suitable for your current state of health.

4. Comprehensive Method:

• When managing diabetes, healthcare professionals adopt a holistic approach, taking into account dietary, lifestyle, medication, and supplementation considerations to create all-encompassing treatment programs that cater to your specific needs and objectives.

5. Responsibility and Assistance:

Healthcare professionals are reliable partners and sources of assistance while you're trying to get healthier. They can provide direction, inspiration, and drive to keep you on track with your supplement and food plans.

Herbal medicines and supplements contribute significantly to the management of diabetes by strengthening insulin sensitivity, blood sugar regulation, and general health. Important vitamins and minerals that are necessary for maintaining good metabolic function and reducing the risk of problems related to diabetes include vitamin D, magnesium, chromium, and omega-3 fatty acids.

More research is required to confirm the efficiency and safety of herbal supplements, including as cinnamon, fenugreek, and bitter melon, which have showed promise in improving insulin sensitivity and blood sugar levels.

Prebiotics and probiotics are essential for maintaining gut health, which is becoming more and more understood to be important for managing diabetes. Prebiotics work as fuel for good gut bacteria, encouraging their development and activity, while probiotics can help regulate the gut microbiome, lower inflammation, and enhance insulin sensitivity.

It's critical to put safety first when adding supplements to your diet and to speak with medical professionals to make sure that the supplements are suitable for your particular needs and objectives. Minimize dangers and optimize benefits by starting carefully, using high-quality supplements, and tracking results over time. Natural therapies include exercise, stress management methods, mindful eating, and herbal teas can support dietary and lifestyle changes for diabetes control in addition to supplements. By addressing all facets of health and wellbeing, these all-encompassing methods enhance general metabolic function and foster long-term fitness. In the end, diabetes management necessitates a whole strategy that involves food adjustments, lifestyle adjustments, medication administration, and, occasionally, vitamin, mineral, and herbal remedy supplements. People with diabetes can create individualized treatment programs that meet their specific needs, maximize metabolic health, and enhance quality of life by collaborating closely with healthcare specialists.

In conclusion, people looking to effectively control their diabetes and advance their general health and well-being can benefit greatly from the use of vitamins and herbal medicines. People with diabetes can enhance insulin sensitivity, lower their risk of complications from the disease, and support blood sugar control by including probiotics, prebiotics, important vitamins, minerals, and herbal supplements in their diet. To be sure that supplements are suitable and helpful for specific health requirements and goals, it is crucial to approach supplementation cautiously, put safety first, and speak with healthcare professionals. People with diabetes can maximize their health and thrive despite the difficulties of the condition by using herbal medicines and supplements with careful planning, close monitoring, and assistance from healthcare professionals.

CHAPTER NINE

MODIFICATIONS TO LIFESTYLE TO AID WITH DIABETES MANAGEMENT

Diabetes management calls for a diversified strategy that goes beyond prescription drugs and dietary adjustments. Modifications in lifestyle are essential for managing blood sugar, lowering the risk of problems, and enhancing general health in diabetics. This extensive book will cover a wide range of topics, including the value of consistent exercise, stress reduction methods, enhancing the quality of sleep, mindfulness and meditation techniques, developing a support network, making long-lasting lifestyle adjustments, and tracking and monitoring results.

The Significance of Frequent Exercise

The foundation of diabetic care is physical activity, which has several advantages for mental and physical well-being. Frequent exercise can help manage weight, lower blood sugar, increase insulin sensitivity, lessen cardiovascular risk factors, and improve overall quality of life. For those who have diabetes, physical activity is essential for the following reasons:

1. Increases Sensitivity to Insulin:

• The body becomes more sensitive to insulin after exercise, which makes it easier for cells to absorb and utilise glucose from the bloodstream for energy. This may lessen the need for insulin or other prescription drugs and help lower blood sugar levels.

2. Reduces Levels of Blood Sugar:

- Exercise causes muscles to absorb glucose more readily, which can result in rapid drops in blood sugar levels both during and after physical activity. Frequent exercise also lowers the risk of hyperglycemia and its related consequences by enhancing long-term glycemic management.

3. Helps With Weight Management

- For people with diabetes, especially those who are overweight or obese, exercise is crucial to managing their weight since it boosts metabolism, burns calories, and builds lean muscle mass. Retaining a healthy weight can enhance insulin sensitivity and lower the chance of complications from type 2 diabetes.

4. Lowers the Risk of Cardiovascular Disease:

- One of the main risk factors for cardiovascular disease is diabetes. Frequent exercise helps strengthen the heart and blood vessels, lower blood pressure, improve cholesterol, and reduce inflammation. All of these benefits help lessen the risk of heart attacks, strokes, and other cardiovascular events.

5. Improves Emotion and Health:

- Endorphins are neurotransmitters released during exercise that increase emotions of happiness and wellbeing. For those with diabetes, regular physical activity can help lower stress, anxiety, and depression, improve sleep quality, and improve overall quality of life.

Aim for at least 150 minutes of moderate-intensity aerobic exercise every week, spaced out across at least three days, with no more than two days without exercise in between, in order to get the benefits of physical activity. Include a range of your favorite activities, like strength training, walking, cycling, swimming, dancing, or other sports. Before beginning a new fitness program, especially if you have any pre-existing medical concerns, speak with a healthcare professional.

Techniques for Stress Management

Stress management is crucial to the management of diabetes since it can have a substantial effect on blood sugar levels and general health. Stress hormones like cortisol and adrenaline are released as a result of prolonged stress, and these hormones can cause weight gain, insulin resistance, raised blood sugar, and an increased risk of cardiovascular disease. Developing excellent stress management skills can assist people with diabetes better control their blood sugar levels and enhance their general health. Consider using these stress-reduction strategies:

1. Breathing Techniques:

• Deep breathing techniques, such belly breathing or diaphragmatic breathing, can assist in triggering the body's relaxation response, which lowers tension and fosters tranquility.

2. Meditation with mindfulness:

• By concentrating your attention on the here and now without passing judgment, mindfulness meditation enables you to more clearly and acceptingly examine your thoughts and feelings.

Frequent mindfulness practice can enhance general mental health and well-being by lowering stress, anxiety, and depressive symptoms.

3. Progressive Relaxation of the Muscles:

• Progressive muscle relaxation helps alleviate physical stress and encourage relaxation by tensing and relaxing various bodily muscle groups. This method can ease muscle soreness and stiffness, lower stress levels, and enhance the quality of sleep.

4. Tai Chi and Yoga:

• Yoga and Tai Chi are mind-body activities that enhance relaxation, flexibility, and balance by combining physical postures, breathing exercises, and meditation techniques. For those who have diabetes, these techniques can promote general well-being, lessen stress, and improve mood.

5. Hobbies and Activities Engaged:

• Taking part in enjoyable hobbies and pursuits can help you decompress, build relationships with people who have similar interests, and function as a pleasant diversion from tensions.

You may enhance your quality of life overall, lessen the negative effects of stress on your health, and more effectively handle the difficulties of having diabetes by implementing stress management practices into your daily routine.

Enhancing the Quality of Sleep for Better Health

Although getting enough sleep is crucial for general health and wellbeing, many people with diabetes experience insomnia and other sleep disorders. Insufficient sleep has a detrimental effect on insulin sensitivity, appetite control, blood sugar regulation, and cardiovascular health, making it an important aspect of diabetes care to address. Here are some ways that people with diabetes can benefit from getting better sleep:

1. control levels of blood sugar:

Getting enough sleep enhances insulin sensitivity and glucose metabolism, which in turn helps control blood sugar levels. Prolonged sleep deprivation raises the risk of hyperglycemia and problems connected to type 2 diabetes by causing insulin resistance, higher cortisol levels, and impaired glucose tolerance.

2. Aids in Weight Management

• Sleep is essential for maintaining energy balance and controlling appetite. Hormones related to hunger, such as ghrelin and leptin, can be upset by sleep deprivation, which can result in an increase in appetite, cravings for high-calorie foods, and weight gain. People with diabetes who prioritize good sleep are better able to control their weight and are less likely to experience consequences from obesity.

3. Enhances Mental and Mood Health:

• Emotional control, mental wellness, and cognitive function all depend on sleep. Chronic sleep deprivation has been linked to mood problems including anxiety and depression, which can make stress worse and have a detrimental effect on managing diabetes. People with diabetes can enhance their mood, cognitive abilities, and general mental health by emphasizing restorative sleep.

4. Boosts Immune Response:

• Sleep is essential for immune system performance, boosting the body's defense against diseases and infections. Prolonged sleep deprivation impairs immunity, making one more vulnerable to infections and inflammatory diseases, which can worsen issues associated with diabetes.

5. Encourages Recuperation and Healing:

• The body goes through vital processes of regeneration and repair as you sleep, which help with muscular growth, tissue repair, and general healing. Restorative sleep is essential for wound healing, glycogen resupply, and recuperation from physical and psychological stress, particularly for diabetics who may be more susceptible to consequences like diabetic neuropathy and diabetic foot ulcers.

Prioritize healthy sleep hygiene habits to enhance the quality of your slumber. These practices include keeping a regular sleep schedule, establishing a calming bedtime ritual, organizing your sleeping space, and avoiding stimulants like caffeine and electronics just before bed. If your sleep problems don't go away, see a doctor to find out what's causing them and look into possible treatments like medication or cognitive-behavioral therapy for insomnia.

Practices of Mindfulness and Meditation

For those with diabetes, mindfulness and meditation techniques are effective strategies for reducing stress, encouraging relaxation, and improving general wellbeing. While meditation focuses attention on a particular object, idea, or sensation to develop awareness and concentration, mindfulness entails paying attention to the present moment with openness, curiosity, and acceptance. Both of these approaches can enhance the quality of life for people with diabetes by assisting them in managing the difficulties associated with their illness. The following are some ways that diabetes patients can benefit from mindfulness and meditation practices:

1. Reducing Stress:

- By encouraging relaxation and lowering the body's stress response, mindfulness and meditation practices can help people with diabetes manage stresses better and enhance their mental health.

2. Blood Sugar Regulation:

- Research has indicated that mindfulness-based therapies can lower hemoglobin A1c levels and enhance blood sugar regulation in diabetics. Mindfulness activities can lower blood glucose levels by fostering emotional balance and reducing stress.

3. Controlling Weight:

- One aspect of mindfulness practice is mindful eating, which promotes people to be aware of their food preferences, hunger signals, and eating habits. Patients with diabetes can control portion sizes, steer clear of emotional eating, and choose better foods by developing awareness and nonjudgmental acceptance of their eating behaviors.

4. Enhanced Quality of Sleep:

- People with diabetes may find it easier to fall asleep and stay asleep if they practice mindfulness meditation, which can help them relax and slow their racing thoughts. People can improve overall sleep hygiene and increase the quality of their sleep by including mindfulness techniques into their nightly routine.

5. Improved Emotional Health:

- People with diabetes can develop a stronger feeling of emotional resilience, acceptance, and self-compassion by engaging in mindfulness and meditation techniques. People can enhance their overall quality of life and more effectively manage the difficulties of having a chronic illness by cultivating a positive outlook and minimizing negative thoughts.

Start with brief guided meditation sessions or mindfulness exercises to begin incorporating mindfulness and meditation practices into your regular routine. To find out more about various meditation techniques and how to apply them in your life, you can use mindfulness applications, online resources, or go to classes or workshops. When engaging in routine activities like eating, walking, or dishwashing, try to be attentive of the present moment by pausing, breathing, and being in the present.

Establishing a Network of Support

Creating a solid support network is crucial for people with diabetes because it offers them social interaction, practical help, and emotional support as they deal with the condition's problems. Family, friends, medical professionals, diabetes educators, support groups, and internet forums can all be considered parts of a support system. The following justifies the significance of a support network in managing diabetes:

1. Psychological Assistance:

- Having diabetes can make daily life emotionally taxing, causing tension, worry, fear, and frustration. A support system offers a secure environment in which you can communicate your feelings, look for approval, and get sympathy and inspiration from people who are aware of your situation.

2. Helpful Advice:

- Monitoring blood sugar levels, following prescription schedules, adjusting to major lifestyle changes, and navigating healthcare systems are all important aspects of managing diabetes. To alleviate the strain of self-management obligations, a support system can provide helpful assistance with things like meal planning, exercise routines, medicine reminders, and doctor's appointments.

3. Knowledge and Instruction:

- A support network can offer helpful knowledge, tools, and educational materials regarding diabetes care, available treatments, ways to modify one's lifestyle, and local resources. People can benefit from each other's knowledge and experiences, stay up to date on the most recent advancements in diabetes care, and make educated decisions regarding their own health by exchanging information.

4. Relationship with Others:

• Having diabetes might occasionally make you feel alone, particularly if you don't have a large support system. Making connections with people who also have diabetes can reduce feelings of loneliness and promote social connection and companionship by offering a sense of understanding, solidarity, and belonging.

5. Drive and Responsibility:

• A support network can offer inspiration, accountability, and encouragement to help people stick to their diabetes control objectives. Having someone with whom to discuss accomplishments, failures, and progress—whether it be a peer mentor, cooking partner, or exercise partner—can help sustain motivation and long-term habit change.

Make contact with friends, family, medical professionals, or neighborhood support organizations for diabetes in order to establish a support network. Additionally, you can join online forums and social media groups dedicated to managing your diabetes, where you can get support, guidance, and encouragement from people who have gone through similar things. Keep in mind that creating a support network requires time and work, so be persistent and kind while establishing deep ties with others.

Making a Change in Lifestyle That Is Sustainable

Making long-term lifestyle adjustments and being willing to stick with healthier routines are necessary for managing diabetes. Make incremental, durable adjustments that fit your interests, lifestyle, and values rather than concentrating on quick cures or extreme measures. Here's how to make a long-lasting lifestyle adjustment to control your diabetes:

1. Establish sensible objectives:

• To begin, make sure your goals are reasonable, attainable, and in line with your skills, preferences, and priorities. To keep motivated and involved, break down bigger goals into smaller, more doable tasks and acknowledge your accomplishments along the way.

2. Put an emphasis on changing behavior:

• Give priority to behavior modification and practices that enhance your general health and well-being rather than just results like weight loss or blood sugar control. Determine the precise steps you can take to optimize the quality of your sleep, reduce stress, increase physical activity, and improve your diet.

3. Locate Pleasurable Activities:

• Pick pastimes and physical pursuits that you look forward to, such as gardening, hiking, dancing to your favorite music, or playing sports. To keep things fresh and avoid boredom or burnout, mix in some freshness and variation to your routine.

4. Exercise Self-Compassion:

• Take care of yourself with kindness and self-compassion as you deal with the highs and lows of diabetes management. Develop a resilient, tenacious, and self-accepting mindset by viewing obstacles and setbacks as chances for learning and development.

5. Seek Expert Assistance:

• Never be afraid to ask for expert assistance from medical professionals, registered dietitians, diabetes educators, counselors, or other specialists. They can offer you direction, accountability, and tailored advice to help you reach your health objectives.

6. Make Modest Adjustments:

• Rather than attempting to completely revamp your routine all at once, concentrate on making tiny, long-lasting adjustments to your living patterns over time. Start small and build on your successes by starting with one or two habits at a time, like include a serving of veggies in your meals or going for a quick stroll after dinner.

7. Remain Adaptive and Flexible:

• Have an open mind and be willing to modify your strategy and course correct as necessary in response to your body's feedback, circumstances, or fresh knowledge. Remain adaptable, flexible, and eager to try out various tactics until you figure out what works best for you.

Keeping an Eye on and Tracking Your Development

It's critical to keep track of your progress in order to evaluate the success of your diabetes control tactics, pinpoint areas that require improvement, and maintain your drive to accomplish your objectives. You can obtain important insights into how your lifestyle choices affect your health and make well-informed decisions regarding changes and adaptations by routinely monitoring important metrics including blood sugar levels, physical activity, nutritional consumption, and mental well-being. Here's how to successfully track and monitor your progress:

1. Maintain a Diabetes Diary:

• Keep track of pertinent information in a diabetic journal or logbook, including blood sugar readings, medication dosages, meals and snacks, physical activity, stress levels, sleep patterns, and mood swings. Analyzing your diary entries over time will enable you to spot trends, patterns, and triggers that could affect how you manage your diabetes.

2. Utilize technological instruments:

• Make use of technological tools like fitness trackers, blood glucose meters, continuous glucose monitors (CGMs), and smartphone apps for managing diabetes. To assist you in making well-informed decisions regarding your health, these technologies can offer real-time data, insights, and feedback. Utilize them to keep tabs on your blood sugar levels, keep track of your exercise, record your food consumption, schedule medication dose reminders, and get tailored advice based on your unique requirements and objectives.

3. Make Measurable Objectives:

• Set quantifiable, precise objectives for managing your diabetes, such as hitting your target blood sugar range, getting more exercise, eating better, managing stress, or getting better sleep. Divide more ambitious objectives into more manageable benchmarks, and monitor your advancement frequently to maintain accountability and drive.

4. Track Your Blood Sugar Levels:

As directed by your healthcare practitioner, check your blood sugar levels on a regular basis using a continuous glucose monitor (CGM) or blood glucose meter. As you monitor your readings throughout the day, take note of any trends or variations. Share your findings with your healthcare team so that your treatment plan can be modified as necessary.

5. Monitor Your Exercise:

- Maintain a record of your physical activity sessions, noting the kind, length, level of intensity, and frequency of physical activity. Establish weekly or monthly physical activity goals and monitor your success over time. As your fitness level increases, progressively lengthen or intensify your activities.

6. Track your food intake:

- Monitor your nutritional intake, including meals, snacks, portion sizes, and the makeup of macronutrients, by keeping a food journal or using a smartphone app. To promote appropriate blood sugar control, pay attention to the quantity and quality of your meals, as well as the amount of carbohydrates you consume. Adjust as necessary.

7. Determine Stress Levels:

- Regularly check in on your emotional and stress levels, keeping an eye out for indicators of stress including weariness, anger, tense muscles, or trouble focusing. To reduce stress and encourage emotional balance, employ self-care routines, stress management approaches, and relaxation techniques.

8. Assess the Quality of Your Sleep:

• Use a sleep journal or tracker to evaluate the length and quality of your sleep, including the time you go to bed, wake up, and any disruptions or problems during the night. Aim for seven to nine hours of restorative sleep each night, and if needed, modify your bedtime ritual or sleeping environment to enhance the quality of your sleep.

9. Consider Your Progress:

• Take some time to consider your successes, triumphs, and difficulties encountered while managing your diabetes. Honor accomplishments, draw lessons from failures, and pinpoint areas in need of development, viewing every event as a chance for personal development.

10. Interact with Healthcare Professionals:

• During routine check-ups or appointments, discuss monitoring data, progress, and concerns with your healthcare providers. In order to create individualized goals and action plans for the best possible management of your diabetes, talk to your healthcare team about any changes in your health status, treatment preferences, or lifestyle habits.

You can obtain important insights into your diabetes management efforts, pinpoint areas for improvement, and make well-informed decisions about modifying your treatment plan or lifestyle choices by routinely monitoring and documenting your progress. Remain proactive, involved, and dedicated to your health objectives. Keep in mind that gradual gains in your general well-being can result from even little adjustments.

Making lifestyle adjustments is crucial for managing diabetes well and has many positive effects on one's physical, mental, and emotional well-being. People with diabetes can take charge of their health and improve their quality of life by implementing regular physical activity, stress management strategies, better sleep hygiene, mindfulness and meditation practices, developing a support network, making sustainable lifestyle changes, and tracking their progress. Never forget that there isn't a one-size-fits-all strategy for controlling diabetes; it's a journey. Try out several tactics, pay attention to your body, and collaborate closely with your medical team to create a customized treatment plan that addresses your unique requirements and objectives. Continue to be proactive, tenacious, and dedicated to managing your diabetes, and acknowledge and appreciate your accomplishments along the way. Despite the difficulties of having diabetes, you may thrive and lead a happy, healthy life if you have commitment, support, and persistence.

CHAPTER TEN

TESTIMONIALS & SUCCESS STORIES IN THE MANAGEMENT OF DIABETES

It may be quite inspiring and enlightening to learn from the experiences of others, particularly when it comes to managing a complicated illness like diabetes. Testimonials and success stories offer insightful, real-life examples of people who have successfully managed their diabetes by overcoming obstacles, changing their lifestyles, and seeing great results. We will examine six fascinating case studies that highlight various methods of managing diabetes, such as dietary interventions, lifestyle changes, and supplementary techniques, in this extensive guide.

Case Study 1: John's Path to Diabetes Type 2 Reversal

John, a 55-year-old man with type 2 diabetes, started a mission to correct his disease after running into issues with pharmaceutical reliance, obesity, and elevated blood sugar levels. John adopted a holistic approach that included regular physical activity, stress management strategies, and nutritional alterations as part of his determined effort to take charge of his health.

Dietary Adjustments:

- John switched to a high-fiber, low-carb diet that was centered on full, nutrient-dense foods such fruits, vegetables, lean meats, and healthy fats. He consumed fewer processed foods, sweetened beverages, and refined carbs; instead, he ate meals that promoted stable blood sugar levels and balanced macronutrients.

Frequent Exercise:

- John made regular exercise a part of his everyday regimen, doing strength training, flexibility, and brisk walking. Most days of the week, he tried to get in at least 30 minutes of moderate-intensity aerobic activity. As his fitness increased, he would progressively up the length and intensity of his workouts.

Techniques for Stress Management:

- John adopted stress-reduction strategies like mindfulness meditation, deep breathing exercises, and relaxation techniques after realizing the negative effects of stress on blood sugar regulation. He placed a high value on hobbies, self-care, and social interactions in order to lower stress and enhance mental health.

Case Study2: Maria's Plant-Based Diet Success

Maria, a 40-year-old woman with type 2 diabetes, found that following a plant-based diet high in fruits, vegetables, whole grains, legumes, and nuts helped her manage her illness very well. Motivated by the advantages of plant-based nutrition in reversing diabetes, Maria drastically improved her health by changing her diet.

Plant-Based Diet:

Maria changed her diet to a plant-based one that consisted primarily of whole, minimally processed foods high in fiber, vitamins, minerals, and phytonutrients. She included a range of vibrant fruits and vegetables into her diet and focused her meals around plant-based protein sources including beans, lentils, tofu, and tempeh.

Blood Sugar Regulation:

By giving priority to plant-based foods with high fiber content and low glycemic index values, Maria managed to stabilize her blood sugar levels and lessen her dependency on diabetes medication. Her general metabolic health improved, her insulin sensitivity improved, and her blood glucose fluctuated less.

Controlling Weight:

- Because plant-based foods typically have more fiber and fewer calories than animal-based foods, switching to a plant-based diet helped Maria reach and maintain a healthy weight. She lost weight steadily and sustainably without experiencing hunger pangs or deprivation, which improved her body composition and metabolic efficiency.

Case Study 3: Mark's Ketogenic Diet-Related Metabolic Change

Mark, a 45-year-old man who was obese and had type 2 diabetes, had a dramatic change in his health after he started eating a ketogenic diet that is high in fat, moderate in protein, and very low in carbohydrates. Mark was first skeptical, but he saw notable changes in his health indices and was able to lose weight in a consistent way by following a ketogenic diet.

Nutrition for Ketosis:

- Mark consumed more healthy fats from foods like avocados, nuts, seeds, olive oil, and fatty fish while adhering to a ketogenic diet that limited his daily consumption of carbohydrates to less than 50 grams. Mark's body transitioned from using glucose as fuel to burning fat for energy by going into a state of ketosis, which led to quick weight loss and enhanced metabolic health.

Regulation of Blood Sugar:

- For Mark, better blood sugar regulation was one of the ketogenic diet's most noteworthy effects. Mark's blood glucose levels were less likely to spike and crash as a result of reducing his intake of carbohydrates and stabilizing his insulin levels. This improved glycemic control and decreased his need for diabetic medication.

Loss of Weight:

- Mark lost a considerable amount of weight while following a ketogenic diet, which helped him get rid of extra body fat and lower his chance of developing obesity-related conditions like metabolic syndrome and cardiovascular disease. Mark found it easier to stick to his diet plan over the long run because of the high-fat, low-carb composition of the ketogenic diet.

Case Study 4: Emma's Intermittent Fasting Experience

Emma, a 35-year-old woman with insulin resistance and prediabetes, investigated the advantages of intermittent fasting as a tactic to enhance her metabolic well-being and halt the development of type 2 diabetes. Emma saw improvements in her blood sugar control, insulin sensitivity, and general well-being after adopting intermittent fasting into her routine.

Protocol for Intermittent Fasting:

• Emma tried a variety of intermittent fasting techniques, such as time-restricted meals, fasting on alternate days, and sporadic extended fasting. She began by following a 16:8 fasting plan, in which she ate all of her meals within an 8-hour window after fasting for 16 hours the previous night. With the help of a healthcare provider, she gradually expanded the window during which she could fast and included longer fasting durations, such 24-hour or multi-day fasts.

An increase in insulin sensitivity

• Emma's insulin sensitivity improved as a result of her intermittent fasting, which helped her cells use glucose and control blood sugar levels more efficiently. Periods of fasting contributed to lower insulin levels and decreased insulin resistance, which in turn resulted in more stable blood glucose levels and a reduced need for diabetic medicine.

Improved Fat Loss:

Emma was able to lose weight and increase her metabolic flexibility through intermittent fasting, which made it easier for her body to alternate between burning fat and glucose for energy. Emma lost weight gradually and sustainably by using her body's stored fat during fasting times. Visceral obesity is a major risk factor for type 2 diabetes and cardiovascular disease.

Autophagy and the Repair of Cells:

• Autophagy, a cellular cleaning mechanism that eliminates harmed or defective components and encourages cellular repair and regeneration, was activated by intermittent fasting. Emma's cells, tissues, and organs were revitalized by this natural cleansing process, promoting her general well-being and long life.

Case Study 5: Using Anti-Inflammatory Foods to Aid Linda's Recoveries

With type 2 diabetes and chronic inflammation, Linda, a 50-year-old woman, set out to restore her health by eating a diet high in whole, plant-based foods and minerals that strengthen the immune system. Linda saw noticeable gains in her overall health and diabetes control by lowering inflammation and promoting her body's natural healing mechanisms.

Anti-Inflammatory Diet:

• Linda developed an anti-inflammatory diet that focused on items including fruits, vegetables, leafy greens, berries, nuts, seeds, fatty fish, olive oil, turmeric, ginger, garlic, and green tea that have anti-inflammatory qualities. She consumed less processed meat, refined sugar, trans fats, and artificial additives—foods known to cause inflammation.

Decreased Inflammation:

• Linda's body showed a decreased overall level of inflammation as seen by decreases in inflammation indicators such as C-reactive protein (CRP) and interleukin-6 (IL-6), which she experienced through dietary modifications. Linda's body became more resistant to oxidative stress, immunological dysfunction, and chronic disease by treating the underlying source of inflammation.

Blood Sugar Regulation:

- Linda's blood sugar levels were stabilized and her insulin resistance was decreased by the anti-inflammatory diet, which made it simpler for her to control her diabetes without taking too many prescription drugs. Anti-inflammatory foods aided Linda's body's capacity to control insulin release and blood glucose levels by fostering hormonal harmony and metabolic balance.

Boosted Immune Response:

Through the use of immune-stimulating foods and antioxidants, Linda enhanced her body's defenses against infections, pathogens, and environmental pollutants. People with diabetes need a healthy immune system since they may be more vulnerable to infections and other consequences.

Case Study 6: David's Narrative of Integrating Supplements and Diets

In order to treat his type 2 diabetes and metabolic syndrome, David, a 60-year-old man, combined dietary interventions with specific supplementation techniques. David saw notable improvements in his quality of life and health markers by correcting underlying dietary inadequacies and improving his food intake.

Nutritional Interventions:

- David adhered to a customized diet that blended aspects of intermittent fasting, low-carbohydrate eating, and the Mediterranean diet. He minimized processed foods, sugar-filled drinks, and refined carbs in favor of nutrient-dense, whole foods such fruits, vegetables, legumes, nuts, seeds, whole grains, lean proteins, and healthy fats.

Specific Supplementation:

David supplemented with essential vitamins, minerals, and herbal medicines that improve insulin sensitivity, blood sugar regulation, and overall metabolic health in addition to making dietary changes. These included vitamin D, magnesium, chromium, berberine, alpha-lipoic acid, and cinnamon, all of which have been demonstrated to be beneficial to diabetics.

All-encompassing Method:

- Rather of merely using medicine to treat the symptoms of his diabetes, David managed his disease holistically, addressing the underlying imbalances and inadequacies that contributed to it. He collaborated closely with medical professionals to track his development, modify his treatment strategy, and enhance his long-term health.

In summary

These case studies demonstrate the variety of methods for managing diabetes and the possible benefits of dietary adjustments, supplementation plans, and lifestyle modifications. Every person's journey is different, therefore what suits one person might not suit another. Nonetheless, people with diabetes can find motivation, inspiration, and useful insights from these testimonies and success stories to support them on their own journey to improved health.

Before making any major adjustments to your diet, workout schedule, or supplements program, especially if you have pre-existing health concerns or are taking medication, it is imperative that you speak with healthcare professionals. People with diabetes can experience significant gains in their health and well-being and regain control over their lives and futures with the help of trained specialists, self-care, and empowerment.

www.ingramcontent.com/pod-product-compliance
Lightning Source LLC
LaVergne TN
LVHW011940180225
804045LV00006B/287